What leading health authorities say about

My Doctor Says I'm Fine ... So Why Do I Fe̶̶̶̶̶̶̶̶̶̶̶̶̶̶
by Dr. Margaret Smith Peet and Dr. Shoshana ̶̶̶̶̶̶̶̶̶̶̶̶

"This book is a synthesis of Western medicine mech̶̶̶̶̶̶̶ of disease and the influence diet and lifestyle have on them with the elegant system of ancient Eastern medicine that allows the body to be its own healer. I strongly recommend this book for its synthesis of these perspectives into a sensible healing program that is owned by the reader."

Jeffrey Bland, PhD, internationally known lecturer, author, and researcher. Author of *Clinical Nutrition, Genetic Nutritioneering,* and over 400 scientific articles. Founder of the Institute for Functional Medicine. President and Chief Science Officer of Metagenics, Inc.

"This book is a valuable contribution for people to have more power in understanding their own healing."

Ted Kaptchuk, OMD, internationally known clinician, lecturer, and teacher. Author of *The Web That Has No Weaver: Understanding Chinese Medicine.*

"A thoughtful and practical guide to Ayurveda, an ancient system of healing with wide ranging scientific possibilities."

Peter D'Adamo, ND, nationally known clinician, lecturer and teacher. Author of *Eat Right 4 Your Type* and *Live Right 4 Your Body Type.*

"The authors take an ancient and complex system of medicine and translate it into a readily accessible set of principles for achieving optimal well being. Similar to the approaches employed by practitioners of Western complementary medicine, they demonstrate the power of basic lifestyle changes to profoundly impact health conditions."

Robert Rountree, MD, nationally known medical lecturer and clinician. Author of *Immunotics: A Revolutionary Way to Fight Infection, Beat Chronic Illness, and Stay Well,* contributor to *A Parent's Guide to Medical Emergencies: First Aid for Your Child, Smart Medicine for a Healthier Child.*

My Doctor Says I'm Fine...
So Why Do I Feel So Bad?

MARGARET SHOSHANA
SMITH PEET, ND ZIMMERMAN, ND

A Summary of Vata, Pitta, Kapha

Vata
THE ENERGY OF MOVEMENT

Dry
Light
Cold
Rough
Mobile
Clear

Pitta
THE ENERGY OF DIGESTION/TRANSFORMATION

Hot
Sharp
Light
Oily
Liquid
Spreading (Mobile)
Fleshy Smell

Kapha
THE ENERGY OF LUBRICATION/ CELLULAR INTELLIGENCE

Heavy
Slow/Dull
Cool
Smooth
Dense
Oily
Soft
Static

 Blue Dolphin Publishing, Inc.
FINE BOOKS FOR ALL AGES

My Doctor Says I'm Fine . . .
So Why Do I Feel So Bad?

My Doctor Says I'm Fine . . .

So Why Do I Feel So Bad?

Margaret Smith Peet, ND

Shoshana Zimmerman, ND

Forewords by
Dr. David Perlmutter, MD
Dr. Vasant Lad, BAMS, MASc

Illustrations by Helen M. Luecke

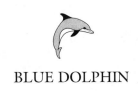

BLUE DOLPHIN

Published by Blue Dolphin Publishing, Inc.
P.O. Box 8, Nevada City, CA 95959
Orders: 1-800-643-0765
Web: www.bluedolphinpublishing.com

ISBN: 1-57733-085-4

Library of Congress Cataloging-in-Publication Data

Peet, Margaret Smith, 1931–
    My doctor says I'm fine-so why do I feel so bad? / Margaret
    Smith Peet, Shoshana Zimmerman ; illustrations by Helen M.
    Luecke.
        p. cm.
    Includes bibliographical references and index.
    ISBN 1-57733-085-4
        1. Medicine, Ayurvedic. 2. Naturopathy. 3. Self-care, Health.
    I. Zimmerman, Shoshana, II. Title.

    R606 .P44 2001
    615.5'—dc21
                                                                2001025365

DISCLAIMER: The information given and discussed in this book is
for research and education purposes only and is not intended to
prescribe treatment.

Printed in the United States of America

10   9   8   7   6   5   4   3   2

This book is dedicated to
Shona Zimmerman and Emma Peet

And to
Michael Dick, Jane Abrams and Zamyat Ventresca

CONTENTS

ILLUSTRATIONS

CHARTS AND TABLES

FOREWORD

HEALTH CARE IN THE UNITED STATES is in desperate need of a change. While annual health care expenditure in America exceeds $1.2 trillion, our rates of cancer, heart disease, diabetes, hypertension, stroke and other chronic debilitating diseases are among the highest in the world. It is time to recognize the profound limitations of a health care system based solely on chemical, surgical and radiation interventions and the patient assessment tools supportive of these therapeutic approaches. As a Rand Corporation fellow was recently quoted in the *Journal of the American Medical Association,* "one-fourth of procedures, and two-fifths of medications could be done without."

Two-thirds of Americans now regularly integrate complementary medical techniques into their health care plans. Indeed the words of Thomas Edison—"The doctor of the future will give no medicine, but will interest his patients in the care of the human frame, in diet and in the cause and prevention of disease"—while perhaps overstated, seem somewhat prophetic.

If you are reading this book, chances are you or someone you care about is suffering from a health-related malady. Likely you were intrigued by the title and are hoping to find the answers not provided by a typical doctor-patient interaction and the laboratory studies which commonly follow. If so, you will be richly rewarded. What follows in these pages is an in-depth, easy-to-understand exploration of the history, science and utilization of an approach to health care that emphasizes not the disease that an individual may have, but the uniqueness of the individual who has the disease. The fundamentals explored in this book are founded upon the oldest of medical texts dating back thousands of years. And yet, these premises remain invaluable not only in unraveling the mysteries of modern diseases but in addition by providing the guidelines for the creation of patient specific health care plans for wellness preservation.

This book helps set the stage for the revolution in health care for which we will all thankfully bear witness.

David Perlmutter, MD
Author: *BrainRecovery.com*
December 2001, Naples, Florida

FOREWORD

IN THIS BOOK, Shoshana Zimmerman and Margaret Peet have written an excellent collective work and a most practical guide for the reader. The first part of the book helps the reader understand what is happening prior to the onset of disease, and the authors open the doors of perception to read the body language in a simple way. One can learn about what is happening within oneself by simply looking at the face in a mirror. By and by, one can observe many interesting things by examining the nails and palms. Each individual finger may be a clue to the person's personality and denotes some unique characteristics. The lines on the forehead can also reveal the present status of health. Similarly, through the eyes, ears, feet and energy pathways one can reach an understanding of personal biorhythm, the life force and the pulse. By knowing the unique individual constitution and current developmental disorder, one will have a guideline for proper diet, lifestyle and cleansing, in order to maintain optimal health.

Both the writers have studied Ayurvedic and Naturopathic medicine. In this book, they have done a unique integration of Ayurveda and Naturopathy, which will be a practical guide for self-healing. The authors have given proper food guidelines as medicine. Doshic imbalance is the root cause of disease and information is given about what to do when a dosha is out of balance. This integrative approach is the medicine of the twenty-first century, a new paradigm that moves beyond the physical.

Ayurveda in the true sense is the mother of all healing systems. It is an all inclusive, holistic science of healing the body, mind and spirit.

Ayurveda goes hand in hand with other medical paradigms. Because one approach alone cannot give the complete picture of a disease, a healer should also study other medical systems. This book entitled *My Doctor Says I'm Fine . . . So Why Do I Feel So Bad?* will be a practical guide for readers.

Dr. Vasant Lad, BAMS, MASc
Albuquerque, New Mexico

ACKNOWLEDGMENTS

THIS BOOK WAS MADE POSSIBLE through the efforts of many people: those who helped us write about complicated concepts in a non-technical manner; those who made it possible for us to have the time and space to write; and those who contributed to the development of Ayurvedic concepts from a Western perspective.

Many friends read our manuscript and offered insightful comments. Some of the readers had no background in Ayurveda or even healthcare issues, others had great expertise. All contributed in major ways. Thanks to Jane Abrams, Jay Brooks, Anne and Joe Edstrom, Gale Halm, Ehrin Johnson, Michele Johns, Helen Luecke, Charles Peet, Kathy Peet, Suzanne Stoterau and Patricia Williams.

In the fall of 1998 we had a contract to write this book but no time to write it and no place to work together. We are indebted to Shona Zimmerman, Shoshana's daughter, and Emma Peet for providing us the time and place. Shona moved to Albuquerque and managed Shoshana's business, making it possible for her to have the time to write. Because of Emma Peet, Margaret's granddaughter, we were able to live next door to one another in Cave Creek, Arizona, from January through June 1999 to write the book. Emma at the age of four months became our daily writing companion. We are also indebted to Heather Murray for opening her home and her heart to us during this time.

Many of the ideas incorporated in this book resulted from a year long collaboration with three wonderful colleagues: Jane Abrams, Michael Dick and Zamyat Ventresca. For almost a year we met weekly for luscious dinners, good wine and much joy and laughter as we brainstormed about ways we could contribute to the growth and understanding of Ayurveda from a Western point of view. We spent precious evenings after dinner in front of a glowing fireplace, sipping chai and exchanging ideas in a way that both sustained and inspired us. The sharing of their friendship and knowledge then and throughout the writing of this book both motivated us and provided us with much joy. We are especially grateful to Michael Dick, an outstanding Ayurvedic scholar, for his work relating everyday qualities we all experience to the process of increasing or decreasing health.

Our thanks and deep appreciation to Hart de Fouw for his critique of the chapter on hand analysis and for his excellent seminars, from which we gained much valuable information.

Our thanks to Paul Clemens at Blue Dolphin Publishing for his helpful suggestions and for giving us editorial freedom to shape the book as we envisioned it. We also want to express our appreciation to Linda Maxwell for her work in laying out the book

Finally, we want to thank Helen Luecke, our illustrator, for lovingly translating our vague words and completely inadequate scratchings into creative and clear illustrations.

We feel special gratitude
for the teachings of the great Ayurvedic sages
who taught us thousands of years ago that

• matter and energy are opposite sides of the same coin

• matter and energy are interchangeable.

And for the teachings of Dr. Vasant Lad,
who helped us to understand the linkages
between the sages and modern scientific thinking.

PART I

WHY DO I FEEL
SO BAD?

CHAPTER 1

HOW YOU GET TO FEELING SO BAD: ENERGY IMBALANCES AND THE DISEASE PROCESS

HAVE YOU EVER HAD THE EXPERIENCE of visiting your doctor because you didn't feel well only to be told there was nothing wrong with you or that you were "perfectly healthy"? Perhaps you were given this information after a battery of tests or after a routine physical exam. In either case, you left the office still wondering why you didn't feel well. Was it all in your head? "If I am so fine," you asked yourself, "why do I feel so bad?" Perhaps you were told that the doctor wanted to keep an eye on things and that you should return for another office visit in a few months. "Keeping an eye on things" meant your doctor wanted to make sure you had not gone from "healthy" to "unhealthy," in an effort to ensure that any disease was identified and treated at its earliest detectable stage.

This kind of experience is quite common, because our Western medical model is not equipped to deal with the disease process prior to the diagnosis of an identifiable disease. That is because the Western model IS a disease model: physicians treat disease. In this book we will introduce you to another medical approach which focuses on what happens in the body prior to the onset of a diagnosable disease.

When you know "something is wrong" and no disease is obvious, you can be left with a feeling of bewilderment. What can you do? What are the options?

Whatever is causing you to feel bad, to feel out of balance, is reflected by your body in ways you can learn to observe. Each kind of imbalance you experience has certain characteristics. You may, for example, have imbalances that can be characterized by the idea of coldness—cold feet and hands, always feeling cold even in a warm room, feeling emotionally cold, etc. Or you may experience the opposite characteristic, too much heat. This can manifest as rashes, infections, fevers, even hot flashes, irritability and anger. It is possible to have both excess cold and excess heat—you can alternate between cold chills and a fever, or have cold hands and feet but also have a hot heartburn from an overly acid stomach.

For you to be able to understand the nature of your imbalances, two things need to happen. You have to develop a conceptual way of looking at yourself, and then you have to know what to look for.

What we see is determined not only by where we look, but also by the questions we ask. Legend has it that the local residents who lived on the tip of South America had a truly unique experience. These "natives" literally could not see the ships of the early explorers approaching. They had no concept that a ship even existed. Not until the explorers got out of the ship and onto the land were they seen.

Some of the concepts we describe may feel as unfamiliar to you as the ships were to the "natives." However, once you "see" them you can immediately apply them to understanding what's happening in your own body.

In this chapter we will introduce you to concepts that may be new to us Westerners, but they have been used for thousands of years quite successfully in the East. In the rest of Part I of this book, we will show you how to look at yourself, physically, in a new way. In Chapter 6 we will help you interpret what you have observed by connecting your markings and other observations with the characteristic symptoms and qualities that are the basis of your imbalances. In Part II we will describe practical steps you can take to bring yourself back into balance. First you will discover ways to deal with specific common problems, and then in subsequent chapters you will learn how to strengthen your immune system. A strong immune system is the best defense against the development of chronic illnesses.

This book is about the processes that create imbalances in our bodies between the time of true health and the onset of disease. Using concepts from Eastern medicine, primarily Chinese and Ayurvedic medicine, there are five interrelated ideas that can help you understand what is happening in your body prior to the onset of disease:

- *The concept of qualities*: how certain qualities such as hot and cold, dry and wet, and light and heavy impact your health.
- *The relationship between qualities and balance*: imbalances can be created by "too much" or "too little" of any quality. For example, "too much" heat can lead to inflammation.
- *The interaction of matter and energy*: the transformation of matter into energy and vice versa is constantly occurring in every human being. Food, for example, is a form of matter we ingest to create energy. Exercise converts more matter into energy. Lack of exercise can lead to weight gain.
- *The nature of body type or constitution*: each person is a unique expression of body type, mind and consciousness. This uniqueness is expressed at the physical, emotional/mental and spiritual levels, together referred to as one's constitution.
- *How constitution is affected by qualities*: "too much" or "too little" of any quality affects all levels of our basic constitution. Too much heat, for example, can make one physically hot, mentally and emotionally agitated, and spiritually exhausted.

Western medicine focuses on the physical, what we call matter. Eastern medicine, in contrast, focuses on life force energy and how that energy is used in ways that either foster or prevent illness. "Life force energy" is energy that sustains all life, and without which life does not exist. It consists of many types of energies, which taken together we call the "life force." The interaction of this subtle life force energy and matter creates patterns of health and illness, and these patterns are reflected by our bodies in specific markings.

With the help of this book you will be able to analyze markings on your face, tongue, hands, nails and even your eyes and ears to find clues about the nature of your personal characteristics. You will learn to recognize indicators of both health and imbalance. In addition, you will learn how life force energy is expressed through the pulse. For us Westerners, this approach may be new and radical, not to mention fun and exciting. In the East, however, it is ancient wisdom. These concepts have been used in India for thousands of years and in China and Japan for almost that long. After your analysis, you will learn a variety of ways to restore balance.

By the time you complete this book:
- You will understand how your state of awareness or con-sciousness affects everything that happens to you, including your health.
- You will understand the relationship between stress, diet, lifestyle and your health.
- You will understand the way life force energy interacts with your physical body to create balances or imbalances in your health.
- You will learn your body's clues about the nature of imbal-ances as they are reflected through specific physical at-tributes and by markings on your face, hands and other locations.
- You will be able to take specific steps to help reestablish balance by selecting from a variety of possible approaches which fit your lifestyle.
- You will know how to strengthen your immune system.

With this information you will be able to begin answering the question that so many of us ask: "My Doctor says I am fine, so why do I feel so bad?" And you will be able to do something about it!

This moment in the history of medicine is exciting. We believe that healthcare is at the cusp of a new era and is in the midst of a paradigm shift to new ways of viewing health as a reflection of the relationship of all parts of an individual—our bodies, emotions, intellect, energy and spirit. The new paradigm has not completely emerged, but we submit that the shift will incorporate the best that medicine from both the West and East have to offer. And it will enable a person to assume some personal responsibility for managing his/her own health in order to create and maintain a healthier lifestyle.

Here in the West healthcare is largely based on technology and the body is viewed in a mechanistic way. Disease is usually assumed to be the result of some sort of outside interference, which ranges all the way from "catching the latest bug" to identifying bacteria, viruses and microorganisms that are linked to specific conditions. While we are aware of unique individual differences, our Western system of medicine cannot anticipate or explain those differences.

In Eastern medicine the sources of health and illness are rooted in how we perceive and experience life—the way we live, including the way we think, feel, act and eat—the way we use our life force. We will study the reasons some individuals have a propensity to "attract" or become a likely candidate for the "successful" development of disease. These individual differences are viewed in relationship to individual constitution and to the concept of balance. While we recognize that external pathogens can make us ill, the emphasis in this book is on examining the way an individual *responds* to the external, including invasion by external pathogens that cause all kinds of infections and illnesses. Two people may be exposed to the same disease. One remains well while the other becomes sick. Why is this the case? Many say that one has a stronger immune system than the other. However, Eastern medicine, particularly Ayurveda, goes beyond that to explain *why* one person is stronger and the other is weaker.

While the diagnostic tools of Ayurveda and Chinese medicine are used extensively, this is not a book about these two systems, but rather a self-help book that you can use to improve the state of your health. Two fundamental approaches are used. The first approach explains how various physical, mental/emotional and spiritual attributes or qualities can create health problems. The second approach guides you through examination of the markings on your body, markings that indicate problems or imbalances that already exist.

That our physical markings reflect the condition of our health may seem a bit radical to some. However, we apply this approach when we look for clues about the condition of a building. There are markings on a building that reveal it needs repair: i.e., peeling paint, wet carpeting, buckled flooring, dampness around plumbing fixtures, drips and leaks. All these are symptoms that there is too much of one quality—wetness. If the owner pays attention, finds the source of the wetness and cuts off the source, in addition to making needed repairs caused by damage from wetness, the building will remain in good condition. Different markings on a building could suggest just the opposite set of prob- lems—dry rot, cracked dry walls, blistered siding. All these markings relate to another quality—dryness. Problems in any building can result from too much wetness or too much dryness. Both are relative terms. It is hard to pin down an exact meaning for "too much." However, when you see a building that is in disrepair, it does not take a giant leap of imagination to realize that significant underlying causes are present.

We can see this same principle applying to the flow of electricity. When there is an excessive amount of electricity flowing to a given piece of equipment, the equipment can become overheated, short-out, or even catch fire. If, on the other hand, there is too little flow of electricity, lights can brown-out and equipment cannot operate correctly. The same processes occur with the flow of life force energy in our bodies.

The Concept of Qualities and Cause and Effect

Most of the time we make lifestyle choices about what we do, think or eat without any particular awareness of the effect those choices have on our health. All of our reactions have certain qualities. Let us look again at the qualities of hot and cold. If we feel too hot, we instinctively look for ways to cool ourselves. When too cold, we look for something to warm us. If we are cool and we want to be colder, we look for something with cooler attributes, perhaps replacing a fan with an air conditioner. In general, we search for like qualities to increase a certain state, in this case to increase coldness. We look for opposite qualities to decrease that state, as in replacing coldness with its opposite, warmth. At any moment we can ask ourselves how we are feeling, cold or warm, and make adjustments to maintain comfort. In this way, we can look at every experience as encompassing associated attributes. Cold is associated with constriction, condensation, tension, tightness, heaviness, slowness. Warmth creates expansion, dryness, relaxation.

In Eastern medicine, an excessive amount of any quality is identified as a cause of imbalance, and prolonged imbalances lead to onset of the disease process. Traditionally, certain qualities have been examined for their impact on a person's health. These qualities are listed below. There may well be other qualities that you find helpful. Traditional qualities that have been used for thousands of years are presented as pairs of opposites:

Hot	Cold	Dry	Oily
Light	Heavy	Slow	Fast
Sharp	Dull	Rough	Smooth, Slimy
Solid	Liquid	Soft	Hard
Mobile	Static	Subtle	Gross
Clear	Cloudy		

These qualities are present around you, and you experience them all the time, at every level of your being—body, mind and consciousness. Any action, thought or event that increases or decreases a given quality has an effect on you. If you eat a large Thanksgiving meal of heavy foods, you will feel heavy, dull and static. You will probably want to take a nap rather than to exercise. If you eat many heavy meals, you will become heavier, perhaps even obese. To lose weight, you will eat foods of the opposite quality, which are light, dry foods. Similarly, any form of agitation will increase feelings of being agitated. Agitation involves the quality of mobility and can come from many sources—your mind running in circles, emotional upsets, too much travel, constant physical movement, bodily restlessness, too much light and gas producing food (such as beans), even too much wind (start checking out whether you are more restless on windy days). To lessen feelings of agitation, of what we would call excessive mobility, you can review what in your life is increasing mobility and begin making changes to bring about the opposite effect. For example, you might learn to control your mind through relaxation techniques, change your form of exercise to a more calming type, eat heavier, non-gaseous producing foods, stay out of excessive wind, etc.

When you start viewing what happens to your body, mind or consciousness from the perspectives of qualities, you begin to have a handle on what you need to do to bring that quality under control, to bring it into balance. You begin tuning into your natural biorhythms and learn to do this moment-to-moment, daily, or seasonally. When you begin to remove the cause, you begin to remove its effects.[1]

The Interrelationship of Body, Mind and Consciousness

In recent years the phrase "body, mind and spirit" has been used to describe total being. In the Western world there are groups of experts to deal with each of these aspects of being. Healthcare practitioners deal with the body. Psychologists, social workers and counselors deal with emotion, and educators deal with the intellect. Philosophers and religious leaders deal with spirit. Graphically this relationship is often depicted as three separate entities:

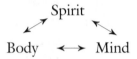

Viewing anyone's state of being as separate entities, however, leads to a false sense of separation. In the Eastern model, body, mind and consciousness/spirit are interrelated, and we prefer to describe these parts of our being as one continuum:

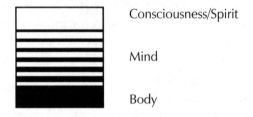

The body is, of course, the physical part of our being. Until recently almost all healthcare concerns in Western medicine focused solely on the body. Then, as stress became recognized as a precursor of disease, it became apparent that one's mental and emotional reactions impact one's health. Almost everyone has had the experience of feeling just fine prior to receiving some devastating news that then led to immediate illness—perhaps an asthma attack, an increase in blood pressure, a migraine, an upset stomach, diarrhea, etc. Similarly, one might feel ill and receive positive news, causing the illness to disappear. This interplay involves a more subtle understanding of health. An even more subtle understanding is the relationship between our state of awareness/

consciousness/spirit and health.[2] Let us look at an example of how the level of consciousness can affect one's health by looking at different ways of viewing a book.

For a person with little awareness a book is a group of pages bound together with a cover. For others a book is a bunch of words on pages. Those with a higher state of awareness, because of the ability to read, might view a book as a series of words that can tell a story or provide information. For still others with an even higher level of awareness, a book can be seen as a physical expression of creative thoughts, insights, emotions and beliefs. At an even more subtle level, a book can be a tangible expression of the author's life force energy through the use of ideas, thoughts, emotions, etc. All these ways of understanding the nature of a book are valid at a certain level. In a similar way, as one's level of awareness or consciousness is increased, one's subtle perceptive abilities increase. At the highest levels a person becomes able to perceive the relationship between subtle beliefs, less subtle emotions, and concrete bodily functions. At this level of consciousness, one's health is seen as the total interplay of one's body, mind and consciousness. Hence an excess of any given quality would be seen to affect every aspect of one's being. For example, the quality of heaviness could be expected to result in an overweight body, a sluggish mind, a heavy depressive emotional outlook, and/or a stagnated heavy state of consciousness. To achieve balance in health we introduce the opposite quality at the appropriate level of body-mind-consciousness.

The Concept of Balance and Life Force

When we feel ill, almost all of us have an intuitive desire to restore our balance so that we feel better. That is what drives us to the doctor in the first place. If in your individual case you are pronounced healthy but you nevertheless feel bad, what are you to do? If you are like most people, you will not just let nature take its course. You will take some action. You might talk to friends, read articles, or consult the clerk at a health food store. Since your doctor does not know what is wrong, you hope against hope the health food clerk can help you out! Pretty soon you have collected a number of products, and you hope some of them will be useful. All this effort is prompted by the intuitive understanding of your need for balance without knowing precisely what to do.

The very word "balance" implies there is a state of being in which the individual is in harmony or in a healthy state. It is a normal state of action and reaction between the systems, tissues and organs of the body. We look at this state as being defined by the relationship of the various constituents of the life force. In Ayurveda, it is understood that the life force is composed of three parts, just as a braid is made up of three segments. These segments are called *vata, pitta* and *kapha.*[3] They are quite complex, and there are subcategories of each, but for purposes of simplification, we will define them as follows:

- *Vata* **is the principle of movement in the body, mind and consciousness.** It is responsible for all physical movements—movement in our internal circulation and elimination systems, movement or changes in our thoughts and emotions and even changes in our state of awareness.
- *Pitta* **is the principle of digestion and transformation.** It is responsible for digestion in the stomach and gastrointestinal tract, in the individual cells and, more subtly, in the "digestion" of one's thoughts and emotions. Well digested thoughts lead to intellectual knowledge; well digested emotions lead to intuitive awareness and self-understanding. When a person feels healthy, intellectually alert and emotionally at peace, personal growth and transformation readily occur. All of these are seen as signs of "good digestion."
- *Kapha* **is the principle of lubrication and organization.** For movement and digestion to take place, lubrication must be present. And since the body is not a mere machine but is intimately changing as a result of inner perceptions and external stimuli, *kapha* maintains cellular intelligence. It is that part of us, for example, that ensures that the heart does the job of the heart and not the job of some other organ or system.

All people must have *vata, pitta* and *kapha* in order to maintain physical existence. Without *vata,* for example, there would be no movement. Even a paralyzed person in a coma must have movement of blood, oxygen and waste products. Without *pitta* there would be no digestion and people would starve. Without *kapha* there would be no lubrication and hence one's arms and legs and other parts of the body could not move. *Vata, pitta* and *kapha* together are called the *doshas*. It is within the *doshas*—within *vata, pitta, kapha*—that the key to balance resides.

Balance and Basic Constitution

Vata, pitta and *kapha* all have specific qualities and characteristics associated with them, which are reflected in the body and pulse. For example, one of the qualities of *vata* is dryness. Common areas that reflect excessive *vata* dryness are the skin and colon. A person can look at the skin and see dryness. Anyone who has been constipated has experienced too much dryness in the colon. In both cases *vata* is too high.

The qualities of any *dosha* can be experienced physically, emotionally, intellectually and even on the level of consciousness. For example, if you feel emotionally dry, you are likely to feel that you have nothing to give, because you are emotionally depleted. When the dry quality of *vata* is present, it can be located in one or more areas. The more areas involved, the greater the imbalance. If you are feeling emotionally depleted, are constipated and have dry skin, you are more out of balance than if you only experience dryness in one or two places. If you are physically, emotionally and intellectually dry, you are more out of balance than if you are simply experiencing physical symptoms such as dry skin or constipation. If you feel totally burned out, as if you have nothing more to give even to yourself, your spirit or consciousness becomes dry. Excess dryness at the level of body, mind and consciousness is a most serious imbalance.

Our *doshas* reflect the qualities that are present in our lives. The following is a breakdown of the qualities associated with each *dosha*:

Vata Qualities

Qualities	Common Manifestations
Dry	Associated with dry skin, hair, lips, tongue and throat, thirst; dry colon, tending toward constipation; "dried up" emotions, feeling emotionally drained.
Light	Reflected in light muscles, bones, thin body frame, light scanty sleep; lightheadedness; skinniness; feeling of emotional spaciness.
Cold	Cold hands and feet, poor circulation; stiff muscles; emotional coldness and aloofness.
Rough	Rough and cracked skin, cracked nails, teeth, hands and feet; cracking joints; rough unrefined movements and mannerisms; rough treatment of others (insensitivity).
Mobile	Fast movements, fast walking, talking, thinking; tendency to do many things simultaneously; restless eyes, eyebrows, hands, feet; unstable joints; multitude of dreams; love of movement, including love of travel; emotional volatility and moodiness, shaky faith, scattered mind; tendency to learn things quickly but also to forget quickly.
Clear	Perceptive, grasping things quickly but forgetting quickly as well; proneness toward emotional emptiness and loneliness.

The lifestyle of a person who is predominantly *vata* will reflect these *vata* qualities. Even the foods that we eat can increase *vata*. Food tastes that are astringent, bitter or pungent all increase the qualities of *vata*. One of the best ways to decrease *vata* is to eat foods that have the opposite qualities: sweet, sour and salty. In the appendices you will find a list of those foods that pacify *vata* and those that increase *vata*. Remember, like increases like. If you eat foods or maintain a lifestyle that abundantly reflects any of the above *vata* qualities, your *vata* will increase and begin to create problems of imbalance that may cause problems long before you have a diagnosable disease. The same is true for the other *doshas*.

Pitta Qualities

Qualities	Common Manifestations
Hot	Associated with good digestive fire; strong appetite; attraction to hot things (food, heat, oral debate); can be hotheaded, willful, determined.
Sharp	Sharp physical features such as sharp teeth, distinctive, penetrating eyes, pointed nose, tapered chin; mentally sharp and alert; emotionally observant but can be critical and judgmental.
Light	Light, medium physical frame; intolerant of bright lights; light skin and hair.
Oily	Soft oily skin, hair, feces; likes to bind or relate to others through control; in excess can become "slippery," manipulative and untrustworthy.
Liquid	Excess urine, sweat and thirst; soft delicate muscles; loose liquid stools; clever at avoiding responsibility.
Spreading (Mobile)	Spreading rashes, acne, inflammation; strong desire for recognition, even fame (spreading one's reputation); can take on too much responsibility, as in spreading oneself too thin.
Fleshy smell	Fetid body odor under armpits, mouth odor, smelly feet; in excess can be attracted to "smelly deals," behavior of questionable integrity.

The tastes that increase *pitta* are sour, salty and pungent. Notice that pungent taste also increases *vata* while salty also increases *kapha*.

Kapha Qualities

Qualities	Common Manifestations
Heavy	Large body frame, heavy bones and muscles; easily gains weight; tends to be practical but in excess can become "heavy handed."
Slow/Dull	Prone to slow digestion, metabolism; walks and talks slowly, tends to learn things slowly and methodically but retains well.
Cool	Digestion is cool, hence sluggish; tendency for cool, clammy skin (especially in humid environments); propensity for colds, sinus and lung congestion, coughs; when excessive, can be quite "cool" under pressure, to the point of seeming emotionally uninvolved.
Smooth	Smooth skin, smooth organs; smooth, calm nature; tendency to be non-threatening and loving; in excess can become too attached.
Dense	Dense, thick skin, nails; large, dense, thick feces; thick abundant hair; dense adipose tissue; slow to change one's mind or position, as in "being dense"; tendency to be emotionally stable; in excess can be insensitive, as in "thick skinned."
Oily	Oily skin, hair, feces; lubricated, unctuous joints and organs; tendency to feel relaxed internally and relaxed with people; in excess can lead to obesity, water retention, or even to a "slippery" individual, one who is unreliable and untrustworthy.
Soft	Soft skin; tendency to be loving, compassionate, forgiving; in excess can become a "softy" easily taken advantage of, unable to establish strong personal boundaries.
Static	Immobile; tendency to love sitting, sleeping and doing nothing.

The dietary tastes that increase *kapha* are sweet, sour and salty. Therefore foods that are sweet, sour and salty increase *kapha*. When out of balance, the desire for sweets, especially sugar, can become overwhelming. Next comes salty oily chips and snacks, as well as fried foods (Kentucky Fried Chicken, anyone?).

Balance and the Qualities of Your Doshas:
Vata, Pitta and Kapha

While all people must have *vata, pitta* and *kapha* to sustain life, we do not all have the same amount of each. There are many combinations, but the most common is for one *dosha* to be prevalent, one secondary, and the third trailing behind the other two. When a person is primarily *vata*, we say that the basic constitution is *vata*. You can determine which *dosha* is dominant in a person by the way he/she exercises, by choices of foods and activities, and by basic lifestyle.

Vata. The qualities associated with *vata* might remind you of fall wind in the high desert: mobile, cool or cold, dry, dispersing, rough, clear and subtle. People who are *vata* dominant are naturally attracted to the tastes that increase *vata*—astringent, pungent and bitter.

Persons who have a basic constitution of *vata* will exhibit many of the charactertistics of *vata* in daily life. Their *vata* is likely to become imbalanced more easily than the other *doshas,* because the very nature of *vata* is movement, and movement implies instability. For example, the *vata* dominant person is likely to become cold easily, have dry and rough skin, hair and nails. That person is prone to be thin as opposed to overweight, and generally has a lean frame and a lanky look (like many models and runners). You can see many *vata* dominant people at the gym working out, and then eating light salads, a smoothie or steamed vegetables. The *vata* qualities reflected in these activities are mobile, light and dry.

The dispersing nature of *vata* can make it difficult for a *vata* dominant person to focus, concentrate or maintain a regular routine. Emotionally, the dry, light, subtle and dispersing qualities of *vata* can affect the person's nervous system so that anxiety, fear, nervousness and tension are easily experienced. In diet, a *vata* type is naturally attracted to dry, astringent, pungent and bitter foods, such as raw or steamed vegetables with almost no oil, sugar or salt in the diet. *Vata* dominant individuals find it easy to be creative, although their creativity tends to come in spurts. Physically, when they become imbalanced, they will initially tend to develop gas and constipation. Almost all *vata* imbalances begin with gas and/or constipation, because *vata* imbalances begin in the colon (the colon or large intestine is considered to be the "homebase" for *vata*). The dry quality of *vata* leads not only to external dryness of the skin, nails and hair, but also to internal drying of necessary fluids, especially those in the colon and the joints.

Over time *vata* dominant people have a tendency, when imbalanced, to develop chronic problems such as osteoarthritis and nervous system disorders such as memory loss and tremors. In the short run they can feel emotionally dry, cold and unnurtured. Excessive dryness or coldness, for example, when accumulated will pour out of the "homebase" and travel to the weakest spot. *Vata* imbalances are often reflected in the bones and nervous systems. Osteoporosis occurs when there is lack of nourishment in the bones and lubrication in the joints. Nervous system disorders can occur when the qualities of cold and/or dry cause constriction along the neural pathways, obstructing the flow of information. When this occurs, in the early stages, a *vata* imbalance can be felt as fearfulness, nervous tension or anxiety. In psychology students are taught to look for the presumed "cause" of fear and anxiety, to look for external events behind such symptoms. In Ayurveda, we might also urge a person to look for causes, but among those causes we would also look for excess *vata*. Often tension, anxiety and fear simply disappear when *vata* is brought back into balance. This is particularly true for non-specific anxiety and fear for which there is no obvious explanation.

Any person can experience high *vata*. However, *vata* dominant individuals experience imbalances of *vata* most easily. Similarly, *kapha* dominant individuals experience *kapha* imbalances most easily and *pitta* types experience *pitta* imbalances most easily. Although a *vata* dominant person will have the strongest propensity to experience the kinds of problems that result from increased *vata*, anyone's *vata* can become out of balance. When it does, they will begin to have *vata* symptoms. This can occur in many ways, especially through eating foods or maintaining lifestyles that provoke *vata*.

Walter is a case of multiple *vata* imbalances. When Walter came to see Shoshana, he was anxious, experienced insomnia and had an extreme fear of becoming poor. He had held a low level, low paying job but had invested wisely. His assets were extensive but his fear of poverty kept him tied to a job that he hated. Every Sunday night or Monday morning (or both) he would become physically ill at the prospect of going to work. While there was no indication of a chronic disease, Walter's life was miserable. Walter was given herbs and a diet that were *vata* reducing. The results were dramatic. Walter was no longer anxious and began sleeping well. In this less fearful state he examined his fear of poverty. He realized that he had been able to create wealth once and if necessary could do it again. He quit the job he hated and moved ahead with his life.

While we who live in the West have not developed the concept of *vata*, we do recognize the existence of *vata* characteristics in certain people. Like the desert wind, we notice that some people are spacey and we call them "space cadets" or "airheads." They display too much *vata*. We admire creative individuals but understand that they have a difficult time being structured and "keeping their feet on the ground." And we know that people who develop chronic debilitating illnesses, such as osteoarthritis and Alzheimer's, usually have dry skin, become easily chilled and easily agitated. All these qualities are associated with *vata*.

The disease process starts with one imbalance and becomes increasingly severe, often resulting in imbalances in all *doshas* before a disease is diagnosed. Therefore, it is important to pay attention to imbalances early and take action accordingly to help prevent more serious problems from developing.

Pitta. *Pitta* is the energy of digestion and metabolism and exhibits qualities connected with fire and water or fluid. A fire is hot, fluid, light and all too mobile if not contained. Heat can feel sharp, especially if one gets too near a flame or touches a hot surface. Fire ashes have an oily quality when touched, as well as an unpleasant odor. The tastes associated with *pitta* are pungent, sour and salty. Hence too much pungent, sour or salty food can increase *pitta*. People who are commonly described as "salty characters" or "sourpusses" have too much *pitta*.

The person whose basic constitution is *pitta* will reflect many of the above characteristics. A *pitta* person will tend to be warm-blooded. In the winter he or she will not need to dress as warmly as *vata* or *kapha* types. As a matter of fact, it is not unusual to see this person wearing a light jacket or sweater when everyone else is bundled up. In the summer, *pitta* people become hot and easily develop sunburn or heat rashes while others around them are feeling quite comfortable. *Pitta* people are naturally attracted to hot foods and warmth-inducing spices such as pepper, mustard, chilis, salt and garlic. Additionally, they are attracted to acidic and sour foods that are heat related: oranges and orange juice, grapefruit, lemons, tomatoes, vinegar and pickles. *Pitta* dominant people also like oily foods, including fried and salty foods, such as potato chips. In the same way as *vata* types, *pitta* people like mobility, because mobility is also a quality of *pitta*. The body of a *pitta* is "medium," meaning it is not the thin, lanky look of a *vata* or the stocky, heavier look of a *kapha,* but somewhere in between.

People who experience too much *pitta* tend to get problems related to heat—rashes, fevers, acid indigestion or inflammations and infections. People with "a fire under them" tend to like to get things done, and hence have an inherent desire to lead and control which can become excessive, leading to tendencies to become domineering, judgmental and angry. Although we have not developed the concept of *pitta* in the West, we all know someone we can describe as a "walking volcano," and people tend to stay out of the path of his/her anger.

Some of the most common problems resulting from excess *pitta* are acute rather than chronic. Inflammatory illnesses are the most frequent—illnesses such as bronchitis, cystitis and even appendicitis. When people suppress the expression of anger, there will be a tendency to increase internal *pitta* related imbalances, especially those related to digestive and liver problems.

Susan is a young woman learning to deal with her anger, especially toward her parents. Susan has accomplished much personal growth with the support of a counselor, and she expresses herself articulately. She is sensitive to and compassionate about the feelings of others and has had a lifelong tendency to turn her anger inward. As a result, when she feels upset and angry, she develops an upset stomach accompanied by nausea. While continuing to work with her counselor, she now also takes herbs and knows which *pitta* provoking foods to avoid, particularly when she is experiencing digestive problems. She is learning to understand the link between her emotional sensitivity, her tendency to suppress anger and her digestive problems.

Kapha. *Kapha* qualities are heavy, dense, solid, stable, smooth, cool, oily and slow with associated tastes of sweet, salty and sour. *Kapha* characteristics are a bit like fudge—heavy, dense and solid. Like fudge, *kapha* is cool, sweet and oily. Physically, a *kapha* person tends to move slowly and methodically. A *kapha* body glistens slightly with an oily sheen and smooth skin that does not easily wrinkle. *Kapha* people are usually patient, loving, compassionate and reliable. Those with excess *kapha*, however, easily develop colds, flus, bronchial and sinus congestion. They easily experience both water retention and weight gain. Excess *kapha* can turn love and compassion into emotional attachment, a fear of letting go of people and possessions. In the West we recognize certain *kapha* characteristics in people we call "couch potatoes," "Earth Mothers" or "Pack Rats." We have created caricatures of "fatty females over 40" who have a hard time adjusting to an empty nest.

Jane has been an "empty nester" for over 10 years. Her three children still live in the same town and she talks to them almost daily. In the past decade, Jane's *kapha* has increased dramatically and she has gained over 80 pounds. She has struggled to learn not to worry about her children, and she recognizes that one of her biggest issues is to learn to let go. Now Jane is beginning to look at how she uses food to meet emotional needs and is learning to change her eating habits. The lowering of *kapha* will also help in dealing with the issues of "letting go."

Much of the healing process for *vata,* and for *pitta* and *kapha* as well, is based on knowledge of the effects of the things we ingest. The qualities of our lifestyle, including our food choices, often match the qualities of the *doshas—vata, pitta* and *kapha*—and what is happening with our health. For example, a person who has the quality of dryness expressed in many aspects of his/her lifestyle will eventually experience problems with health that are based on excessive dryness. A person who lives in the desert, seldom drinks liquids, does vigorous exercise that leaches out liquid from his/her system, eats dry foods and has very little emotional satisfaction is bound to experience excess dryness. It would be no surprise for such a person to initially develop skin problems, nervous anxiety and constipation and more complicated problems over time unless the imbalance of dryness is corrected.

Balance and Basic Constitution

When anyone is experiencing symptoms of illness, even in the absence of a diagnosable disease, the system is out of balance due to the presence of excess or insufficient qualities. Analyzing qualities inherent in symptoms and relating the qualities to *vata, pitta* and *kapha* give insights into the nature of imbalances and provide the basis for correcting them, whether related to lifestyle, exercise, diet, emotional patterns, etc. However, there is a precise way to determine the type and location of an imbalance. The method involves identifying a person's basic constitution and then identifying how much his/her current state differs from the basic constitution.

It is known in the West that one's genetic code is determined at the point of conception. This code provides our genetic blueprint for life, even giving rise to inherent propensities for attracting certain illlnesses. In the East another kind of code is also created at the point of conception. It is one's life force energy code and is a reflection of the patterns of *vata, pitta* and *kapha* at conception. Like DNA, this code is an inherent part of the individual for life. As previously mentioned, most people are dominant in one *dosha*, secondary in another, and the third trails behind. If *vata* is dominant, *pitta* secondary, and *kapha* third in line, we would express it as *Vata 3 Pitta 2 Kapha 1* ($V_3P_2K_1$). In contrast, if *pitta* is primary, *kapha* secondary and *vata* third, we would express it as *Pitta 3 Kapha 2 Vata 1* ($P_3K_2V_1$). These relationships are reflected in one's pulse.

The relationship of the *doshas* at the point of conception defines the individual constitution. However, as we become imbalanced through the process of living, we develop our current state of *vata, pitta* and *kapha*. This too is reflected in the pulse. For example, a person's basic constitution might be *Vata 3 Pitta 2 Kapha 1* ($V_3P_2K_1$) while their current state is *Vata 4 Pitta 3 Kapha 1* ($V_4P_3K_1$). This would tell us the person has too much of some of the qualities associated with *vata* and *pitta*. Changes need to be made to bring those qualities back into balance. When that is achieved, the current pulse pattern will match the basic constitution, and the person's state of balance and health will be restored. Remember, the pattern of *vata, pitta* and *kapha* is not limited to the body. It is also reflected through one's entire being—body, mind and consciousness—including the pulse.

The impact of lifestyle and diet on one's constitution can be so great that a person's dominant *dosha* may be relatively balanced while the other *doshas* are severely imbalanced. This type of imbalance is illustrated by the lifestyles of June and Mark.

June's basic constitution is *pitta* dominant. Her current state is *vata* dominant. June's lifestyle is *vata* provoking. While in her early forties, June became obsessed with aging and wanted desperately to look younger and remain attractive to men after her divorce. She limited her food intake drastically and was sometimes anorexic. She exercised compulsively, doing aerobics, skiing and biking, all of which jarred her joints and dried out her body. She frequently had joint aches and pains. Her skin and hair were dry despite the use of expensive shampoos and moisturizers. Her daily routine was non-existent—no routine other than to see kids off to school and generally be there when they returned. June was independently wealthy and did not work. As a result, she was free to dabble in many things but tended to lose interest easily. Her behavior became quite dramatic. She moved quickly, as if darting from here to there. June's speech was so rapid it was sometimes hard to keep up with her. She lived in a state of nervousness and anxiety and was particularly concerned about her appearance—wrinkles, dry hair and skin.

June understood that her basic constitution was *pitta,* but her imbalances were almost all a result of *vata,* because her lifestyle was extremely *vata.* As her fear increased, she became less and less willing to look at underlying reasons—high *vata* and questions about the purpose of her life. Like almost everything else in her life, Ayurveda was treated as a fad. In the course of Ayurvedic treatment, she panicked when *vata* started to decrease and she became calmer. "What do I want to do when I grow up?" was a question that then plagued her. Rather than using her newly acquired calmness to help her gain insight, June retreated back to the "safe" area of "busy, busy, busy" frantic activity.

June demonstrates how a person of another constitution, *pitta* dominant in this case, can become out of balance in another *dosha,* in her case *vata.* In addition, her case demonstrates that *vata* imbalances are the easiest to correct clinically but the most difficult to correct practically, because people with high *vata* find it difficult to get into and stay in a regular routine. The volatile, changing nature of *vata* makes compliance difficult. *Vatas* hate consistency and routine. However, those who make changes can make rapid progress in cases that have not yet developed into chronic illnesses.

In contrast, Mark suffers from high *kapha* even though his constitution is *vata* dominant. He has been diagnosed with polycystic disease by his allopathic physician and has had surgery to remove cysts from his kidneys. Cysts have *kapha* qualities. They are dense, cool, solid and hard but smooth. The kidneys process fluid. Mark is quite concerned about his health and was willing several years ago, after his surgery, to make necessary changes to strengthen his immune system and either slow down or prevent the growth of further cysts. He faithfully follows an Ayurvedic lifestyle, taking herbs, making dietary changes, exercising, relaxing, and meditating. Mark is tested every six months and so far there have been no more cystic growths. The severity of his health problems and his personal commitment to his own health motivated him to establish and follow a new lifestyle. He feels better, has more energy and is no longer so susceptible to getting every little "bug" that comes along. This has occurred despite the fact that the disease process was well advanced in Mark's body. People with high *kapha* can readily implement systematic changes, because the nature of *kapha* supports slow gradual change.

Decreased Doshas

Most of the time we discuss the *doshas* in terms of increased qualities, because the prevalence of increase is the basis of almost all imbalances. However, it is possible to have decreased *doshas*. When present, decreased *doshas* indicate serious conditions that are reversed with extreme difficulty, if at all.

Signs and Symptoms of Decreased *Doshas*		
Vata	*Pitta*	*Kapha*
Loss of sensation	Hypothermia	Extreme dehydration
Speech impairment	Anorexia (complete lack of appetite)	Sensation of internal burning
Stupor	Cold extremities (such as frostbite)	Atrial flutter/fibrilation
Shock	Coma	Extreme dryness, thirst dizziness, palpitation
Comprehension impairment		Sudden loss of blood pressure

A state of decreased *dosha* is an acute condition that generally needs hospitalization. These conditions are different from chronic conditions with similar symptoms because of their sudden onset.

Determining Your Basic Constitution and Your Imbalances

You may ask how you can determine your basic constitution. The most accurate way is through pulse diagnosis. The next most accurate way is by carefully and thoroughly observing bodily features, food and lifestyle preferences. There are many "tests" in various Ayurvedic books to help a person identify constitution. However, these tests more accurately indicate current state than basic constitution. In addition, the tests are racially skewed to reflect the qualities of Caucasians. For example, a blue-eyed Caucasian who is thin with dry skin and somewhat dry, frizzy hair is generally a *vata*. There are many African-Americans, Native Americans, Asians and others who are *vata* dominant but do not have these characteristics.

So how do you tell? One way is to study the characteristics that you had as a child and compare them to your qualities now. Are they the same? Have you always been thin and lanky, active physically and mentally, hating to sit still, and wanting to jump from one thing to the next? Did you tend to be forgetful or to be a daydreamer or full of nervous energy? Did you prefer dry foods such as dry cereal and raw veggies or salads. Are your patterns the same now? If so, you are likely to have a *vata* dominant constitution.

Similarly, if *pitta* was dominant in your childhood, you might well have liked leading and organizing, being in charge and getting things done, with others or by yourself. Your childhood ailments were likely to have been heat related, including fevers, rashes, sunburns, chicken pox and indigestion. Your food preferences might have been toward salty or sour, hot or spicy foods.

The *kapha* dominant child wants to be well-liked, popular and sensitive to the needs of others. If your basic constitution is *kapha,* your shape even as a child would have tended to be a little wide and generally stronger than your *vata* or *pitta* playmates. *Kapha* children are attracted to sweet, salty and oily food and can easily become overweight. They tend to like wheat and dairy products such as pizza, hamburgers, fried chicken, french fries and desserts, especially ice cream.

Most adults can easily compare current lifestyles to their childhood to determine constitution. However, this is much more difficult for anyone who grew up on fast food and lots of TV, because such food choices and sedentary lifestyle create *kapha* imbalance at an early age.

Even if you are never positive of your basic constitution, it is still possible to identify your imbalances by the kinds of qualities, symptoms and body markings you have. Note your symptoms and match them to the qualities listed under *vata, pitta* and *kapha.* If the symptoms are strong enough to be bothering you, they are almost always in need of decrease, so introduce more of the opposite in your lifestyle, including diet, to reestablish balance. You will be amazed at the results that can be achieved by changing the qualities in your life. It may take more time in the case of *kapha* imbalances or when any *doshic* imbalance has become severe, but the results can be dramatic, or sometimes subtle. You simply one day become aware that the formerly irritating symptom is no longer present.

The apparent subtlety of this process was brought home to Shoshana in a follow-up appointment with a woman who was not happy with the results of one month's efforts. She went through each symptom one by one with the client and quite surprisingly almost all of them were gone. The client had only been aware of the symptoms that were continuing to cause her problems. Suddenly she stopped in mid-sentence and exclaimed, "I just realized that my shaking has stopped. My arms and hands have been shaking for 25 years and they don't shake anymore!" Clearly, to assess your progress it is helpful to keep a list of your symptoms and check them off one by one as they disappear. Otherwise, you might only be aware of the problems that still remain and become discouraged. And look for possible benefits you had not even expected. They might not be as dramatic as the above example, but they may very well be significant enough to make a qualitative difference in your life.

It is important to learn how to look at your body and be able to tell if any or all of the *doshas* are out of balance. Remember that for any constitution any *dosha* can be imbalanced. According to Ayurveda, all diseases start with imbalances in the *doshas*. When a *dosha* is imbalanced, you will experience the qualities of that *dosha* as symptoms. Long before any disease develops, there may be "non-specific" symptoms, which are clues to determining the imbalances in your *doshas*. Additionally, as you learn the basic markings on your body, you will have further information about the nature of your imbalances. And then you will learn steps to reverse the imbalances and restore health. How easily the imbalance will reverse will depend in part on how far along you are in the disease process and how diligent you are in making needed lifestyle changes.

CHAPTER 2

MIRROR, MIRROR ON THE WALL: A CLOSE LOOK AT YOUR FACE

YOU ARE ABOUT TO BEGIN ANALYSIS OF YOUR FACE for clues about your health, personality, and any imbalances you may have in your *doshas,* your *vata, pitta* or *kapha.* As we describe the different steps of analysis, keep in mind that no one observation indicates a pattern. An individual mark or observation is a clue, nothing more. It does not necessarily signify that you have a disease. A single observation that is not confirmed by other observations on the tongue, ears, eyes, hands, nails or pulse may simply be an indication that you are at the early stages of an imbalance. It is a *pattern* of clues that is the most helpful. If for example you have the indications of an imbalance of heart energy on the face and tongue, you need to pay attention. If these indications also exist on the fingers, ears, nails and eyes, you need to pay more serious attention. And if you are lucky enough to have a pulse diagnosis done by a well-trained practitioner, and heart energy imbalances are in the pulse, it might be wise to see your allopathic medical doctor for testing.

> **In this chapter you will learn to:**
> - **Relate these markings to health and personality traits**
> - **Observe key markings on your face**
> - **Relate those markings to balances/imbalances in your major organs and tissues**
> - **Relate those markings to common changes in the *doshas,* in *vata, pitta* and *kapha.***

At first you may question the usefulness and accuracy of this approach. It is not scientific in our Western sense. However, it is important to recognize that our current level of medical analysis is based on internal, rather than external, indicators. Blood, urine, feces and spinal fluids are examined. Instruments are inserted and we are pricked, x-rayed, scanned and explored through various medical devises. All of these are used to discover markers of disease. Prior to the development of analytical tests and equipment it was common for physicians to diagnose in part by external observations.

In Eastern medicine, complex diagnostic systems have been developed around external observations and pulse diagnosis. These systems have been successfully used for thousands of years. That Western medical science makes no great use of these systems does not mean the information they provide is inaccurate. Quite the opposite. Nothing lasts for thousands of years unless it has merit. Our current scientifically based medical model incorporates new information and insights continuously, expanding our knowledge of how the body functions. At the same time we have begun to experience a little humility about some of the emerging limitations of science-based medicine. For example, we are beginning to understand that overuse of drugs has led to drug resistance and the emergence of bacterial infections that are impervious to drug treatment. Additionally, large scale scientific studies of heart disease, diabetes, and cancer are indicating that fundamental improvements in health are best made through lifestyle changes which include diet, exercise and relaxation techniques. The question then becomes which kind of lifestyle changes can a person make that will be most beneficial. Using the analytical tools we provide to understand your external markings or clues along with application of concepts of *vata, pitta* and *kapha* can provide you with enormous insights and workable approaches to restoring your own health.

The combination of observation and self-knowledge about your non-specific or specific symptoms will yield useful information. Just be careful to avoid the pitfall of most first year medical students who see all symptoms in themselves and fearfully conclude they have all kinds of diseases. We suggest you observe, record your observations, and look at the patterns. There is a personal checklist at the end of this chapter to assist you. Then, and only then, prepare an interpretation of which *doshas*—*vata, pitta* or *kapha*—are out of balance. Study the qualities of your imbalances and then select the antidotes to reestablish balance that are outlined in Part II of this book. Enjoy the journey you are about to take, and use what you learn wisely.

General Facial Characteristics: The Head

We will begin by examining sections of the face and what to look for within the sections. Then we will identify common facial markings and their associated meanings, and provide case study examples based on actual or composite cases.

The face below is divided into three sections. The forehead area provides indicators that are associated with the nervous system. It is in this section that we discover markings that indicate, for example, whether a person is anxious or relaxed, and whether any anxieties are related to material, psychological or spiritual concerns. In the mid-section we view the circulation systems and their related organs, heart, lungs and kidneys. The markings in this area relate to circulatory conditions. The bottom section indicates the status of the digestive system. Intuitively, we recognize the validity of these facial areas. Cartoonists rely on this information. A worrier is drawn with forehead lines. Someone who is angry and about to "pop a vessel" is drawn with a red, often swollen looking face. Those with stomach upsets and digestive problems have frown lines on the chin.

Face by sections

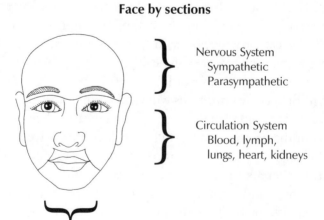

Digestive System: Colon, small intestine

The drawings below show a healthy, youthful looking face and its opposite. In addition to the markings, it is helpful to look at the color, tinge and texture of facial skin.

Healthy and unhealthy faces

Healthy: Few markings   Unhealthy: Many markings

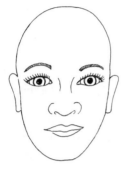 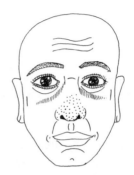

The color, texture and markings on the face
all give clues about personal imbalances.

Look carefully at the color and tinge of your face. Regardless of skin color, is there a reddish tinge? A yellowish tinge? A whitish pallor? Are there any broken veins or capillaries on the face, especially near or on the nose? What is your skin texture? Is it rough or smooth? Oily or dry? Spotted with pimples and acne? *Vata* dominant people tend to have rough, dry skin with bumps. *Pittas* tend to have reddish or yellowish skin, and *kaphas* have a lighter more whitish pallor. These same characteristics are exhibited by American Indians, Asians, African Americans and other people of color, although the variations are subtle and may require careful observation to ascertain.

Forehead Lines

Look at your forehead. Do you have lines? If so, how many? Are they deep or shallow? Solid or broken? Horizontal or vertical? Most people have light forehead lines in their early twenties if not before.

Forehead lines

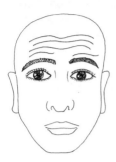 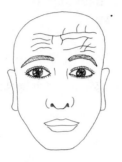 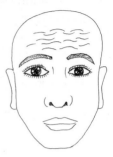

Unbroken
forehead lines

Vertical & horizontal
broken forhead lines

Horizontal broken
forehead lines

However, *kaphas* who are calm, cool and collected or *kaphas* with thick skin often do not have these lines. *Kaphas* who are not in a state of *vata* imbalance do not generally have excessive sensitivity in the nervous system. Things "slide off their back" more easily than is true with the other types.

If you have forehead lines, check out the number, the relative depth of each, and whether they are solid or broken. Most people with lines will have three of them. Some will also have lines above their eyebrows. The lines are thought to reflect your basic orientation to life and provide information about doshic imbalances. In both Ayurveda and Chinese medicine, the top line reflects a person's values and spiritual interests. The center one represents personality and ego, the lower line a person's relationship to practical, earthly matters, including work and finances. Look at the number and length of your horizontal forehead lines and at the nature of these lines, their depth, whether they are broken and whether they are wavy.[1]

Unbroken lines: If all three lines are unbroken, distinct and strong, a person tends to have a balanced view of life. He/she is likely to experience little conflict between the spiritual and practical and feel self-confident in most situations. Three deep, clear lines indicate general good health and sound judgment. Anyone who is lucky enough to have such lines, and whose diet, exercise patterns and lifestyle are compatible with their constitution, is likely to have a healthy and meaningful life.

Broken lines suggest potential problem areas. A person with a broken bottom line may have conflicts on the physical level, perhaps in work or finances. A person with a broken middle line may have problems related to personality or ego. A person with a broken upper forehead line may exhibit problems on the level of values or spiritual concerns.

Broken lines also indicate areas of intermittent change in health, sometimes for better and sometimes for worse—which most of us experience.[2]

Wavy lines: People whose forehead lines are wavy tend to experience frequent changes in health and are prone to unclear or fuzzy thinking. They tend to have a hard time making decisions or finding a direction in life. Changes mark their lives—job changes, partner changes, changes in location, changes in ideas or even religious affiliation. The grass may always look greener on the other side.

Missing lines: A missing line or lines may simply be the forehead of a *kapha,* or it may indicate a significant blind spot, or both. Every human being has some blind spots in life, some more, some less. People with blind spots may remain unconscious of the spots or learn to be aware of them, becoming concerned about the involved life areas. The location of a missing line has significance. For example, a person with a missing middle line is likely to have little regard for those who emphasize personality issues. Those with strong middle and lower lines tend to have strong personalities, to seek leadership or business positions, and to avoid spiritual matters. Those with only a spiritual line tend to have high ideals but may be impractical. Those with only the personality line tend to have strong personalities and must guard against egotism. They may be indifferent to possessions except as status symbols that boost their sense of superiority. Those with only the material line tend to look for material security.[3]

Occasionally a person has two short but distinctive lines above the eyebrows. These are intuition lines. People with these lines have the ability to assess the character of others. In addition, they have worked diligently to develop their personal levels of awareness and self-honesty.

At the end of this chapter there will be a chart to help you analyze your own face.

Lines Between the Eyebrows

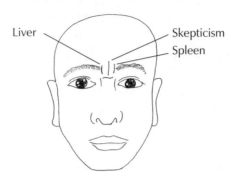

Lines between the eyebrows

It is common to observe individuals with vertical lines at the base of each eyebrow. The one on a person's right side represents the liver and the one on the left the spleen. In Ayurveda the liver is viewed as an organ for cleansing whose function can be negatively affected by diet and anger. A deep liver line is a clue that there is an imbalance in the liver energy.

That observation in and of itself does not indicate whether a liver imbalance has begun to manifest on the physical level. Additionally, it does not indicate whether an imbalance is *vata, pitta* or *kapha*. One of the earliest indications of manifestation on the physical level is tenderness under the rib cage on the right side where the liver is located. The *vata, pitta* or *kapha* nature of an imbalance can be determined by accurate pulse analysis long before any physical symptoms are present. In lieu of that, however, you can rely on other clues. For example, a person who is overweight, has high cholesterol or has an enlarged fatty liver is likely to have a *kapha* imbalance. In contrast, a person who otherwise displays *vata* imbalances and has a liver line should consider the possibility of hardening of the liver, which may lead to cirrhosis. A *pitta* with a liver imbalance may develop mononucleosis, jaundice, hepatitis or other inflammatory conditions.

A vertical line on the left is related to the spleen. Physically the spleen is the largest of the lymph organs and produces lymphocytes that protect the immune system. The spleen also removes toxins and dead blood cells and platelets from the blood. Most physical problems with the spleen involve its enlargement and/or rupture. The major causes of spleen problems are infections and inflammations, which are *pitta,* and anemias and cysts, which are *kapha.*[5]

The spleen energy is related to the integration of body, mind and consciousness. Those who feel at war with themselves can experience such internal stress that their spleen's ability to integrate, protect and cleanse is compromised.

While liver and spleen lines are quite common, sometimes there is a third line located midpoint between them that tends to be longer than the other two. This line indicates a propensity to be questioning or skeptical. People with this line seldom take things at face value. They are the "show me" types. While initially skeptical, once they have analyzed a situation carefully, they are likely to trust their conclusions, in part because they know they have "thought it through." There are, of course, exceptions.

The relationship between forehead lines and personality character-istics is exemplified by Cheryl and Robbie.

Cheryl has three solid unbroken forehead lines and a deep and long vertical midcenter line. Those who know her describe her as solid—interested in the integration of her values, personality and practical aspects. She is initially skeptical, but once she analyzes a situation and reaches a conclusion, she can be relied upon to follow through with any commitments she has made. Robbie, in contrast, has three broken forehead lines and a deep and long vertical midcenter line. Robbie is filled with ideas that he cannot implement, is described as extremely scattered by those who know him, and cannot be relied upon for anything. Robbie is always skeptical but his analysis and conclusions mean nothing. He can be described as "blowin' with the wind."

Undereye Markings and Bags

The areas under the eyes are fascinating to study. The color, puffiness, depth and shape of the lines all provide information about the functioning of the kidneys and adrenals, including the body's level of hydration or dehydration. Dehydration is quite common in the West

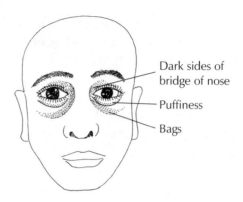

Undereye markings

because of addictions to caffeine in the form of coffee, black tea, certain soft drinks and chocolate. Caffeine stresses the adrenals, kidneys and spleen, and is diuretic. In addition, few people drink sufficient water. Over time those who are dehydrated develop darkness on the upper nose areas next to the eyes which spreads downward and under the eyes. Not only is this viewed in Ayurveda as a sign of dehydration, it is also seen as an indicator of a stressed immune system. Problems can be caused either by dehydration or excessive hydration. Some people think they absolutely must drink eight or more glasses of water per day. We have seen clients who drank one to two gallons of water per day. If a person is thirsty and kidney energy is strong, this causes no problem. But if kidney energy is weak, it is like whipping a tired horse. The more that is drunk, the worse the condition. The entire body can become puffy.

Janice drank at least a gallon of water a day, thinking it was good for her. As a nurse she was quite busy and postponed urination for hours. Her skin when touched felt like a sponge and left deep indentations when pressed. Through simply learning to drink when thirsty and urinating at the first urge, she lost over 10 pounds in water weight and the sponginess of her skin disappeared.

Bags: In the bag area other markings are also of note. There can be small pimples between the eye and the bag areas. This shows the presence of too much mucus within the tiny renal arteries. When these pimples harden or dark dots develop in the pouches below the eye, kidney stones may be developing. Sometimes the presence of fat appears as yellowish deposits under the skin. Cholesterol and fat build-up in the kidneys can lead to stones.[6]

Puffiness: If puffiness under the eyes appears, primarily from the eyelid hair follicles to any circles under the eyes, adrenals are likely to be involved. If the puffiness is on the lower side of the eye circles, salt and water retention are indicated. Salt contracts and causes the renal arteries to close, weakening the kidney and causing high blood pressure as well. The darker the color under the eyes and the deeper the bag lines the stronger the indication of low kidney energy. Dark brown bags indicate a serious condition. The darker the eye bag area, the more so. Darkness indicates that the kidneys are becoming exhausted and unable to purify the blood, hence a build-up of waste within the kidneys and in the blood.[7] We have never seen any person who has had a kidney removed or had a kidney transplant who did not have dark brown circles under the eye on the side of the body of the removed kidney.

Infants and small children with bluish bags under their eyes are becoming increasingly common. Donna and Timmy, who are both three, are examples. Donna has been raised on iced diet drinks, salty chips, candy and fast food. Each day she drinks at least one Coke, has a bag of chips and is almost always given candy as a treat for being a "good girl." Lunch is usually fast food. Donna has bluish coloring and undereye bags from dehydration and immune system problems—and she is only three! Timmy's mother breastfed him when she was addicted to cocaine and rarely ate anything other than junk food. Timmy became addicted to cocaine through the breast milk. He not only has bluish eye coloring and eye bags, but also developed a hypersensitive nervous system. Timmy now lives in a loving environment with good nutrition and emotional support. While the bluish marks and bags are disappearing, he still has an overly sensitive nervous system and must be given herbs to function calmly and sleep well.

In Eastern medicine the kidneys are the storehouse of the body's life force and the site from which the life force is distributed throughout the body. As such, any imbalance in this system will in time affect other bodily systems, organs and tissues. Depletion of this life force energy can result from many factors: stress, excessive work, anxiety, excessive sex, poor diet, inadequate exercise, and living a lifestyle outside nature's natural rhythms (such as working all night, living almost exclusively indoors under artificial lighting, eating only processed foods, etc). The role these factors have on the kidneys and adrenals is generally understood. However, excessive sex as a source of kidney exhaustion is a concept almost unheard of in the West.

In Eastern medicine, the kidneys are regarded as the seat of sexual vitality as well as the storehouse of the body's life force. Engaging in excessive sex can exhaust and damage the kidneys and also the bladder. Who has not heard of someone who came back from a honeymoon with a bladder infection? What constitutes "too much" sex? Stay aware of the pouches under the eye. During times of unusually active sexual activity, if you begin to see darkness or swelling in the eye pouches, a period of rest is needed.

Joan was thrilled with her newly found love and they shared a marvelous honeymoon in the Caribbean. Her sex life was what one might expect from a honeymooner in love. But she returned from her honeymoon with both cystitis and a weakened immune system that led to a strep throat, not to mention physical exhaustion.

The Nose and Cheeks

  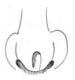

| Pitted & bulbed: heart problems | Broken blood vessels: liver imbalance | Cleft: heart energy imbalance | Indentation: lung energy imbalance |

The nose gives clues about conditions of imbalance in the heart and lungs. Those who have a large, pitted, bulb shaped nose at the tip are prone to heart problems. If there are broken blood vessels present on the nose or side of the face on the cheeks, liver imbalance is also a possibility. Alcohol, allergies and clogged arteries can cause nose and cheek capillaries to expand and break. When the sides of the nostrils are permanently red and swollen in appearance, hypertension may be developing. Sometimes there is a cleft near the middle or bottom of the nose, an indicator that the right and left sides of the heart are not well coordinated.[8] Perhaps there is a heart murmur. A cleft is to be distinguished from a simple indented line. A mere surface line indicates the presence of hemorrhoids, usually internal.

Lung energy is connected to the grooves on the side of the nose. Deep groves where the lower nose area attaches to the cheek indicate weakness in the lung energy. This marking is common in the West where many people are shallow breathers, taking breaths that only fill the upper lungs. Some of the life force in the body comes from the intake of *prana* through breathing. Therefore, the failure to breathe deeply has widespread consequences. Western medicine focuses on the intake of oxygen through the breath. Insufficient oxygen causes problems in the functioning of all cells, those of the brain in particular. In the digestive tract, insufficient oxygen slows the digestive process, and in the brain it impedes mental clarity and memory. In Ayurveda, oxygen is said to be the food of *prana*. Deep breathing and physical exercise can improve the intake of both *prana* and oxygen in the body. The groove at the side of the nose is also connected to the bronchi. Excessive consumption of dairy, sugar, foods with chemical additives or foods to which one is sensitive or allergic can cause this area to become red, inflamed, and congested with mucus.[9] Most of us have experienced a red nose when we come down with the "flu," a serious cold, or severe allergy reactions.

Ben had deep grooves on the sides of his nose as a young man. He was a smoker and also worked around toxic chemicals. He worked in the building trades and walked a great deal up and down stairs in his work, but that form of exercise alone was not enough to compensate for his weak lung energy. In his thirties and forties Ben became susceptible to bronchitis and pneumonia. He then developed emphysema and had to take disability retirement. He did stop smoking but otherwise has taken no action to strengthen his lung energy. He has had one lung collapse in his retirement, has a difficult time breathing, is constantly short of breath, and faces having to use an oxygen tank if or when his lungs deteriorate further. His nose grooves are quite deep.

The nose groove area is associated with the large intestine (colon). The body's energy paths, or meridians, run throughout the body in orderly patterns. The meridian for the large intestine ends at the side of the nose. When toxins begin to build up in the colon (the large intestine), there will be an accumulation of mucus in the pores at the side of the nose and, in more severe cases, along the side of the cheek following the meridian. When the colon does not eliminate properly, the colon energy moves along the meridian to the nose and sinuses, resulting in mucus and congestion in the sinuses and lungs. Just for fun, study the drawings below that indicate the primary meridians in the face and then compare these lines to your own experience. Have you experienced rashes, acne, pimples, eczema, headaches or pain along any of these lines? If so, look for other symptoms of imbalances that may be found elsewhere on your face, tongue, eyes, hands, ears, etc. There will be a more detailed discussion of the meridians in another chapter.

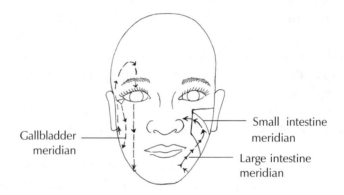

Gallbladder meridian

Small intestine meridian

Large intestine meridian

Facial meridians

The size and shape of the nostrils is a reflection of the size and shape of the lungs. Wide, flaring nostrils indicate large lungs with a great capacity for oxygen. Large lungs are a sign of strength. They represent the body's ability to breathe in large quantities of the life force. Those who are able to take in a great deal of *chi* or *prana* are able to have a great

Nostril size

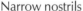

Narrow nostrils   Small nostrils   Large nostrils   Uneven nostrils

impact on life through pursuit of their personal goals. When a person's ability to take in *prana* is small, his/her ability to give out is also small.[10] However, the possession of large nostrils does not guarantee adequate intake of *chi* or *prana*. If one's lifestyle is sedentary and breathing pattern shallow, lung energy may be weak, in spite of contrary indications.

Roger has deep grooves on the sides of his nose but also has large nostrils. He is committed to his work and allows almost no time for rest or to cultivate close relationships. Roger does not exercise. His lifestyle is sedentary and his breathing is shallow. Whenever Roger gets a cold or flu, it tends to settle in his lungs. He frequently suffers from bronchitis or asthma.

When one nostril is small and the other large, the lung on the side of the small nostril will usually be smaller than the one on the side of the large nostril. Nostrils that are too small or too long and narrow make for diminished lung capacity. When breathing or aerobic exercise is undertaken for an extended period of time, subtle changes in the shape of the nostrils are observable.

Jean had a lifelong problem of shortness of breath that was unrelated to exercise. Even with extensive body conditioning, she could not walk up a hill without breathing heavily through her mouth. Her nostrils were long and thin. Recently she had surgery to increase the size of her nostrils and noticed immediate changes. She now rarely experiences shortness of breath. More surprising to her was a change in the shape of her nostrils. They have become wider and more open. While still long, they no longer resemble narrow slits.

There are lines that extend from the nostrils to the sides of the mouth that indicate colon conditions. The deeper the line, the stronger the imbalance. A deep line near the top by the nose is related to the ascending colon, midline relates to the transverse colon and bottom to the descending colon.

Colon markings

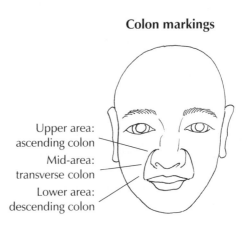

Upper area: ascending colon

Mid-area: transverse colon

Lower area: descending colon

The Mouth

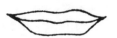 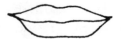 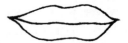

Thin upper lip: problems assimilating nutrients, weak stomach

Full, medium size mouth: good digestion

Enlarged lips: chronic digestive problems, prone to stomach upsets, constipation and/or diarrhea

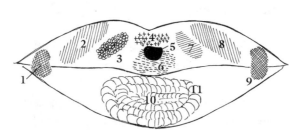

1. Left kidney
2. Left lung
3. Spleen
4. Thyroid
5. Heart
6. Stomach
7. Liver
8. Right lung
9. Right kidney
10. Small intestines
11. Large intestine

The mouth indicates the condition of the digestive tract. The upper lip reveals the condition of the stomach and other organs, the lower lip the condition of the small intestines and colon (the large intestine). If either or both lips are swollen and have perpendicular lines, there are problems with the digestion. If the upper lip line is distinct and well defined, a person has a naturally strong stomach. If the upper lip becomes obscured or shrinks, the stomach is weakening. It is common to see shrunken, undefined upper lips in older people, indicating lack of nutrient assimilation and degeneration. Often these people have mouth odor as well, caused by fermentation in the stomach.

The midsection of the lower lip shows the condition of the small intestines. Often there are white patches and sometimes red or blue patches in this area, indicating a lack of circulation in the small intestines. A dark red or purplish patch indicates more serious blood stagnation, and a change in diet and more rigorous exercise are called for. The bottom lip also shows the strength of the colon (large intestine). When the lip is swollen, there is often a chronic bowel problem, either constipation, diarrhea or both. Red or purplish patches on the lower lip also indicate stagnation in the colon. Red or brown dots may indicate the presence of hemorrhoids or ulcers. If the lower lip also has vertical lines and the lip is swollen, the condition is usually hemorrhoids.

The sides of the mouth indicate the condition of the energy of the duodenum. If the sides become cracked, it may be because of the presence of excess bile attempting to digest excess fat. Too much bile can back up, enter the stomach, and create ulcers.[11]

For an interesting and eye-opening exercise, pick up any women's fashion magazine and analyze the models' facial markings. You will notice that what is now being portrayed as beautiful is actually a reflection of ill health. How many of the models reflect kidney and adrenal problems? Almost all of them. How many have swollen lips? Almost all. These affects can be produced by makeup and silicon injections. The point is that what is being portrayed as beautiful and what many people are trying to accomplish with their looks is in fact unhealthy, as unhealthy as the anorexic bodies of many of these models. Perhaps the time is nearing when an organization can be formed of Mothers and Dads Against Sick Anorexic Models. The need for such an organization is at least as strong as the one that led to Mothers Against Drunk Driving.

The Sides of the Mouth and the Chin

On either side of the mouth one can often find an indentation in the skin which indicates fluctuating energy, a sign of pancreas imbalance. A severe imbalance can result in hypoglycemia or diabetes, both resulting from improper sugar metabolism.

Next to indentations on either side of the mouth, there may be dimples or lines that are connected to imbalances in the energy of the reproductive organs. We often view women with dimples as especially attractive. However, they are quite likely experiencing PMS or other reproductive system problems. Men with dimples may also have reproductive system difficulties.

Under the lower lip many people have a line that looks like a frown line. This line indicates unresolved grief and sadness, often at an unconscious level. With the fast pace of life here in the West, it is not at all uncommon to see this line. People have little time to resolve the proliferation of emotions that arise with constant demands and the bombardment of information. Emotional suppression can result in this "frown line" without any conscious recognition of the problem. On the physical level, this line is also related to the reproductive system.

Lower face and chin lines

Line: reproductive system problems
Line: pancreas, fluctuating energy
Curved line: grief or sadness / reproduction
Broken lines: prostate, zinc deficiency
Dimple: frustration

Sometimes broken lines can be seen in the chin area of men, indicating an imbalance in prostate energy. Those who have such lines should also check for white spots on their fingernails for indications of zinc deficiency. Prostate cancer and zinc deficiency go together. Men with broken lines should have prostate exams on a schedule recommended by their physicians.

Finally, a dimple mark in the center of the lower chin indicates frustration. This is a common marking with people who hate their jobs or other aspects of their lives, but feel there is no manageable escape from their situations. When the mark is hereditary, it indicates a propensity to experience frustration. For an example of this marking in a well-known person, look at the face of John Travolta.

Examine your face for each of the areas mentioned above using the facial diagram. As you learn to check markers in other areas, look for those that are related to the possible problem areas you have already identified. Wherever there are similar indications in the other areas—on the tongue, nails, eyes or elsewhere—imbalances are stronger. When you discover imbalances, you have the opportunity to make lifestyle changes or to ignore your observations, at your peril. When changes are made, the results can be seen by changes in the markings. On the face the markings change gradually, on the tongue they change more quickly.

Unhealthy face

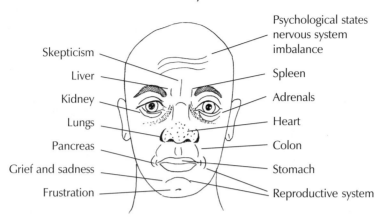

Skepticism
Liver
Kidney
Lungs
Pancreas
Grief and sadness
Frustration

Psychological states
nervous system
imbalance
Spleen
Adrenals
Heart
Colon
Stomach
Reproductive system

Lynn's face reveals multiple problems. Lynn had a stressful job, was raising children by herself and had no support system. Her forehead lines were deep and broken, she had liver and spleen imbalances, pancreas imbalances and severe dysmenorrhea with her menses. She could see no way to keep up with all the demands on her time and carried both a high level of frustration and grief and sadness about her social isolation. Her spiritual growth was important to her and, as she became more trusting and less fearful, over time the forehead lines disappeared, as did the liver and spleen lines. After her children were grown and left the nest, Lynn was able to overcome her social isolation and began to enjoy life immensely. Through both counseling and spiritual work, her former fearfulness was replaced by greater self-confidence as well as greater trust. She still has pancreas imbalances so the indentations on the sides of her face are still present. She now experiences little grief and sadness and the line on her chin has become faint. The frustration dimple has disappeared. Lynn is pleased with the changes in her life. With fewer line markings she even looks younger!

Your Personal Checklist

If you have taken notes up to this point, review them and fill out the checklist below to begin to understand the nature of your own imbalances.

Personal Checklist	
Do you have lines on your forehead? Are there three lines? Are any of them broken? If so, in which line?	Suggests nervousness. A broken line suggests a difficult area that requires extra attention. Top line: ideals and values Middle line: personal psychology and ego Bottom line: practical "earthly" affairs, including career and finance
Do you have vertical lines at the base of either eyebrow?	Right line: liver energy imbalance, possibly suppressed anger Left line: spleen energy imbalance, possibly weak immune system
Do you have a center line?	Indicates skepticism
Are there baglines under your eyes?	Suggests kidney energy imbalance
In the area between your eyelid and the bagline, is there: • puffiness • yellowish spots • brown spots	 Indicates adrenal stress Indicates buildup of fat in kidney tissue May be developing kidney stones
Is there discoloration or dark tones from the nose downward along the bag line?	Suggests dehydration
Are there deep grooves at the sides of your nostril?	Could be problems with your lung energy or lungs
Is the tip of your nose reddish and bulbous, as if swollen?	Check for heart energy imbalances that can lead to arteriosclerosis (clogged arteries) or heart disease

Are there any broken capillaries along the sides of your nose or along the cheeks?	Suggests the presence of liver imbalance and build up of toxins in the liver
Are the nostrils the same size? Large or small?	Related to lung problems and imbalance
Are there lines from your nostrils to the edges of your mouth? Is the line any deeper in one section or the other?	Related to colon Top: ascending colon Middle: transverse colon Lower: descending colon
Is your top lip shrunken?	Relates to stomach and small intestines
Is the bottom lip swollen?	Relates to colon assimilation problems
Are there vertical lines in the upper or lower lips?	Relates to digestive problems
Do you get sores on the sides of your mouth?	Relates to overly acid stomach
Do you have any clogged pores, pimples, eczema or acne?	Look for location along major organ Meridian points on face
Is there a "frown line" under your lip on your chin?	Emotionally related to grief and sadness Physically related to reproductive system
Do you have broken chin lines?	Can indicate prostate imbalance in males and difficulties with ovaries in females
Are there lines on either side of your mouth?	Suggests pancreas related energy fluctuation
Are there dimples on the sides of your mouth?	Suggests hormonal reproductive imbalance
Do you have a dimple in the center of your chin?	Suggests a high level of frustration

CHAPTER 3

LOOK AT YOUR TONGUE:
IT'S FOR MORE THAN JUST TASTING

WHILE WE ALMOST ALL LOOK AT OUR FACES at least once a day and brush our teeth in front of a mirror, tongues are not looked upon as an item of beauty, so chances are you don't know what yours looks like. We hope that is about to change.

The tongue is an extraordinary diagnostic tool. It has been valued for its diagnostic insights by Eastern medicine for thousands of years. Doctors in the West before World War II always asked their patients to stick out their tongues, and some still do. However, today Western physicians depend more on lab analysis.

The tongue occupies the floor of the mouth. It is constructed of interlacing masses of skeletal muscles held together by connective tissue. The tongue contains mucous and serous (watery fluid) glands, many small pockets of adipose cells and the sensory receptors that allow us to taste our food. In addition to making speech possible, the tongue mixes food with saliva and initiates swallowing, the first step in the digestive process.[1]

Because the tongue is a mucous secreting organ, the outer layer or coating of the tongue is highly sensitive and capable of rapid change. Any change in our health, especially one that involves mucous production in our bodies, affects the skin around the mucous membranes, making it either crack or discharge mucus. Because of the mucous secretion of the tongue, this organ reveals much about the present condition of our health.[2]

Although pulse diagnosis can be much more precise in giving detailed information about our health, the tongue gives reliable general indications of both chronic and acute conditions. The tongue, combined with reading of the face as outlined in Chapter Two, gives abundant information.

Ted Kaptchuk, a Doctor of Oriental Medicine with whom Margaret studied, spoke of an elderly Chinese physician who "described the tongue as a piece of litmus paper that reveals the basic qualities of a disharmony. Many signs may be interpreted only when the entire configuration can be seen, but the tongue interpretation is always essential. It is often the clearest indication of the nature of a disharmony and its pattern, reliable even when other signs are vague and contradictory."[3] The tongue quickly reflects changes in current conditions.

Many tongue characteristics are significant: the shape (thick, thin, long, short), the color (red, yellow, white, purplish, brown, black), the flexibility (stiff, flabby, contracted, swollen), the tone (trembling, still, fluctuating). From examination of the tongue one can read the state of *vata*, *pitta* and *kapha*, plasma, blood and digestive fire. When aggravated by *vata*, the tongue is dry, rough and cracked. When aggravated by *pitta*, it is reddish in color with sores or ulcers and a burning sensation. When aggravated by *kapha*, it becomes coated, white and slimy. The tongue of an anemic person loses its normal color and becomes pale. When digestive fire is impaired, the tongue becomes coated with toxins. The tongue is a window to the state of digestive fire and points the way to future health. Examination of this important organ reveals the totality of what is happening in the body.

Reading Imbalances on the Tongue	
Vata	Dry, rough, cracked, inflexible, stiff, contracted, trembling, pale
Pitta	Reddish in color Sores or ulcers Burning sensation
Kapha	Coated, white, slimy, swollen, flabby
Anemia	Pale
Low digestive fire	Coated with toxins

In this chapter you will learn how to:
- Identify tongue shapes for *vata, pitta* and *kapha* constitutions
- Learn the significance of color, flexibility, tone and coating
- Understand the significance of basic tongue markings
- Analyze *doshic* imbalances on your own tongue
- Compare the information you learn from your tongue with that inferred from the facial markings

The Body of the Tongue

In tongue analysis, a distinction is made between the body of the tongue (the tongue itself) and its coating (outer layer). The color of the body of the tongue is the single most important aspect of tongue diagnosis. To observe the color of the tongue itself, be sure to look beneath any coating. If the coating is thick and heavy, lift the tongue and observe the color of the underneath area. The color of the tongue body almost always reflects the true condition of the patient, irrespective of temporary conditions such as those resulting from daily digestion, recent physical exertion or emotional upset. It is the body of the tongue that indicates long term or chronic conditions.

What is the appearance of a "normal," healthy tongue? We put quotes around "normal" because very few people have a healthy tongue. However, most newborns have a healthy tongue, which is a pale pink. Little Emma had a healthy pink tongue at birth. When she was two months old, a white coating appeared on the surface of her tongue. When her mother, who was breastfeeding her, gave up dairy and eliminated caffeine, Emma's tongue cleared.

The body of the tongue can be various shades of red with varying degrees of moisture. A "normal" tongue is pale red or pinkish and somewhat moist, due to healthy circulation, abundant blood supply and *prana*. It looks like healthy flesh. In fact, a healthy tongue has been described as having the appearance of a piece of raw chicken from which the skin has been removed. It is moist and pink, with no unusual markings except perhaps a thin transparent coating. The ancient Chinese medical texts say that the heart opens into the tongue and the condition of the heart and the blood are reflected through the tongue.

The normal, fresh, pale red color of the tongue body indicates that the tongue is receiving an abundant supply of heart blood.[4]

The healthy tongue should also have what the Chinese call "spirit." Its appearance should be vital and vibrant. The body of the healthy tongue is supple, neither flabby nor stiff. It is not cracked, does not tremble or quiver and is neither swollen nor thin. The normal coating is thin and transparent, which indicates the normal functioning of digestion. The tongue should also be slightly moist.[5]

A pale tongue is less red than a normal tongue and indicates a blood supply that is deficient in red blood cells, causing anemia, a cold condition. A red tongue is redder than a normal tongue and points to excess heat in the body due to an imbalance of *pitta*. A scarlet tongue indicates a more extreme heat condition, with *pitta* having entered the deeper levels of the body. A purple tongue points to stagnation of circulation and can perhaps indicate problems with the heart.[6]

Let's look at the pale tongue in a bit more detail. A pale tongue body can range in shades from slightly pale to nearly white in extreme cases. A pale tongue indicates a condition of internal cold in the body, caused by either deficiency of red blood cells leading to anemia, or lack of blood supply to the tongue caused by stagnation in circulation. If stagnation affects peripheral circulation, a person may have cold hands and feet or perhaps a cold nose. If stagnation is in the central circulation affecting the deeper organs, a person's digestive fire may be affected, leading to problems with metabolism and proper digestion of food. A pale tongue body can usually be classified as *vata* in Ayurveda, because *vata* is cold. However, a pale tongue can also be *kapha*. In Chinese medicine, a deficiency of red blood cells is called "deficiency of blood," and when that is present the tongue is dry as well as pale. When stagnation is present, the tongue is wet as well as pale. Blood deficiency is more common in women and stagnation is more common in men. "Other clinical manifestations of (blood deficiency) include numbness, dizziness, impaired memory, a dull and pale face, insomnia, scanty periods in women, and a choppy pulse. Other clinical manifestations of (stagnation) include chills, loose stool, a bright white face, and a deep, weak pulse."[7]

Look at your tongue. Is it pale and dry? Or is it pale and wet? If you answer "yes" to either of these questions, make a note of it. A pale tongue indicates that you should take food and herbs that have a warming effect to lessen the body's internal cold and provide internal warmth. For example, ginger tea will warm and stimulate the body.

A tongue that is redder than a healthy tongue indicates excess heat in the body, high *pitta*. Inflammation is an indicator of high *pitta*. If the entire body of the tongue is red, it indicates heat throughout the body. If only parts of the tongue are red, only various organs and systems are affected. A red tongue is usually dry, since excess heat dries the body fluids. However, if stagnation is present, the tongue may be wet as well as red. A bright red tongue indicates that you should take cooling and moistening food and herbs to lessen the heat.

When observing your tongue in a mirror, indirect natural sunlight is best. If you must use artificial light, incandescent is better than fluorescent, unless the fluorescent is full spectrum.

Reading the Body of the Tongue	
Normal healthy tongue	Pale red Somewhat moist Looks like healthy flesh Vital and vibrant appearance (spirit)
Pale tongue	Vata or kapha imbalance Internal cold Anemia Cold hands and feet (peripheral circulation) Low digestive fire (central circulation)
Red tongue	Pitta imbalance Excess heat in the body
Scarlet tongue	Extreme heat condition, Pitta
Purple tongue	Stagnation of circulation May indicate problems with the heart

The Shape of the Tongue

The shape of the tongue body includes not only its physical shape but also its motility (ability to move). A normal tongue shape is neither too thin nor too swollen, and is soft and supple without being flabby. The tongue tapers toward the tip. It can be extended easily and neither trembles nor quivers.[8] The normal shape and size for each constitution—*vata, pitta* or *kapha*—is slightly different. We will discuss each in detail.

A thin tongue is often seen in a person with a *vata* constitution. One of the qualities of *vata* is dry, and the tongue of a *vata* person is often dry and has a shrunken appearance. Fluids give fullness to the tongue. If a thin tongue is pale as well as dry, the cause may be due to a deficient supply of blood, leading to anemia. A thin tongue that is red and dry indicates excess heat in the body, *pitta*.

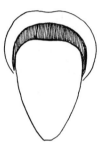

Vata tongue: thin, small, usually dry, pointed tip

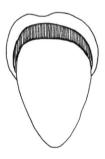

Pitta tongue: medium, long, pointed tip

The usual shape of a healthy *pitta* tongue is thin but with a thicker base than the *vata* tongue described above. When a *pitta* tongue is long and reddish, it indicates a tendency to heart problems. Other clinical manifestations of a long reddish tongue include insomnia, mental restlessness, redness of the face, dryness of the mouth, thirst, mouth ulcers, dark yellow urine and a rapid pulse.[9]

The tongue shape usually associated with a *kapha* constitution is fuller in width and thickness than the tongues described above. A *kapha* tongue easily fits in the mouth without the sensation of fullness associated with a swollen tongue.

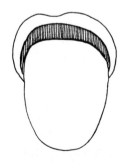

Kapha tongue: large, wide, thick, rounded tip

Abnormal Tongue Shapes

Many problems spring from imbalances that are reflected on the tongue. Tongues may be swollen, thick, stiff, trembling or contracted.

Swollen: A swollen tongue, usually a *kapha* condition, gives the feeling of filling the entire mouth. The thickness of a healthy tongue reflects a normal supply of blood and fluids. If a tongue is swollen, it means that excess fluids are distorting its size. This condition may be caused by stagnation. If the color of the tongue is a healthy pink, the swelling may be caused by low digestive fire and may be accompanied by a sense of abdominal fullness and hypothyroidism.

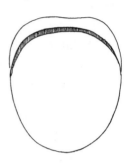

Swollen tongue

Stiff: A stiff tongue has lost its flexibility and resembles a piece of wood. This condition may manifest with characteristics associated with both *vata* and *pitta*. It may be caused by emotional factors, such as anxiety, fear, insecurity, inflexibility or obsessiveness. A stiff tongue may indicate a serious condition, especially if it is accompanied by slurred speech. A tongue's dexterity is directly related to the condition of the heart. A strong heart reveals itself in good enunciation. Slurred speech often indicates some type of cardiovascular problem.[10] A stiff tongue always reflects a disharmony in the body. If you have a stiff tongue, it would be wise to see your allopathic doctor.

Trembling: A trembling tongue when extended is usually associated with an imbalance of *vata*, due to insufficient *prana* (the life force) to regulate proper movement. A trembling tongue is also an indication of anxiety due to high *vata*.

Contracted: A contracted tongue that cannot be stretched out may indicate a serious condition. When the color of such a tongue body is pale or purple, internal cold is probably the cause. A swollen, contracted tongue may indicate excess fluids or mucus. If such a tongue is red and dry, it is a sign that *pitta* has dried the body fluids. See your doctor.

Look at your tongue in a mirror. What shape is it? Is it thin, dry or shrunken in appearance? Is it thick? Does it tremble? Is it swollen or stiff? Long or short? Make a note of your observations. Use the individual tongue analysis chart at the end of the chapter.

The Shape of the Tongue Body

Thin tongue	Usually *Vata*, Often dry Shrunken appearance
Thin tongue with thicker base	Usually *Pitta*
Fuller in width and thickness	Usually *Kapha*

Imbalances Reflected on the Body of the Tongue

Swollen tongue	Usually a Kapha condition Feeling of filling the entire mouth Excess fluids distorting size Stagnation or low digestive fire
Thin, pale and dry tongue	Deficient supply of blood, leading to anemia, Vata
Thin, red and dry tongue	Excess heat in the body, Pitta
Long and reddish	Tendency to heart problems Insomnia Mental restlessness Redness of face Dryness of mouth Thirst Mouth ulcers Dark yellow urine Rapid pulse
Stiff tongue	Vata and Pitta condition Loss of flexibility May be caused by: —Emotional factors —Condition of heart if accompanied by slurred speech
Trembling tongue	Vata imbalance due to lack of Prana or anxiety
Short or contracted tongue	Serious condition Pale or purple: internal cold Swollen: excess fluids or mucus Red and dry: Pitta has dried body fluids

The Coating of the Tongue

Now you will want to look at the coating on your tongue. First, look at the areas that are most coated. Then look at the color of the coating.

As indicated in the previous section, the tongue body indicates longstanding or chronic conditions. The coating gives information about present or acute conditions. The color of the coating can range from watery and clear to thick and yellowish or even darker. The coating (surface layer) is often the result of the digestive process and can reflect the state of the gastrointestinal tract and digestive fire.

The coating may cover the entire surface of the top of the tongue body or it may be confined to patches. It can vary in thickness, color, texture and general appearance. In a healthy individual, it is thin, transparent and moist, and the tongue body can be seen through it.[11]

White coating: A white coating covering the entire body of the tongue indicates toxins in the gastrointestinal tract. Wataru Ohashi, a well known teacher of shiatsu in New York City with whom Margaret studied, says there are two basic causes of white coating on the tongue: 1) excessive amounts of fat, cholesterol, dairy products and baked goods in the diet, which lead to congestion in the system and blockage of blood circulation; and 2) overeating.[12]

A thick layer of white coating on the tongue indicates stagnation in the digestive tract, leading to accumulation of undigested food and toxins. In the body's attempt to eliminate excess accumulation, the tongue becomes coated.[13] The total absence of coating—a bald, dry tongue—indicates serious internal dehydration.

Yellow, dark brown or black coating: The coating on the tongue can also be yellow, dark brown or black. Yellow coating indicates a problem with the liver or gallbladder and suggests excess bile in the blood. Darker colors may indicate the presence of fungus or kidney involvement, and may suggest a serious problem. See your doctor.

Other coatings: A coating that is puddled with moisture is a sign of excess fluids, due either to a condition of cold in the body caused by insufficient *pitta* or by excess *kapha*. A coating that is dry is a sign of deficient fluids, perhaps caused by high *vata*, or excessive heat, caused by high *pitta*. A greasy coating that appears thick and oily is a sign of mucus and excess oil or fat, both of which are excess *kapha* conditions. The tongue's coating can also be an indicator of acid or alkaline conditions. Whitish coatings may be caused by alkalinity in the body and thick yellow or brown coatings may be caused by excess acidity.

Look at your tongue in the mirror. Does it have a white or yellow coating? How thick is the coating? How much of the tongue does it cover? Is the tongue dry or wet? Are canker sores present on the tongue or in the mouth?

Reading Imbalances on the Coating of the Tongue	
Thick white coating	Stagnation in digestive tract
Bald, dry tongue	Serious internal dehydration
Yellow coating	Problems with liver or gallbladder
Dark brown or black	Fungus Kidney involvement
Coating puddled with moisture	Excess fluids —Insufficient Pitta —Excess Kapha
Dry coating	Deficient fluids —High Vata —High Pitta, excessive heat
Greasy coating	Kapha —Mucus —Excess oil or fat
Thick yellow or brown	Excess acidity
Whitish coating	Excess alkalinity

Organ Locations and Markings on the Tongue

Different areas of the tongue body are related to different organs of the body. Although both Chinese and Ayurvedic medicine assign locations on the tongue to specific organs, there are slight differences in the two systems. In this book we will use the organ locations and interpretations outlined by Dr. Vasant Lad in *Ayurveda: The Science of Self-Healing*.[14]

Tongue analysis

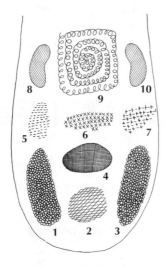

1. Left lung
2. Heart
3. Right lung
4. Stomach
5. Spleen
6. Pancreas
7. Liver
8. Left kidney
9. Colon / small intestine
10. Right kidney

Referring to the tongue map above, let's look at some specific markings, such as depressions, lines, cracks and colors, for additional information about what is going on in our bodies.

Center line: The first marking is the line down the middle of the tongue. This line is related to the spine and the locations of deeper parts of the line indicate problem areas. If the line is deep toward the back of

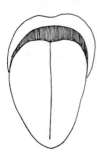

Tongue: center line – emotional well-being, spine shape

the tongue, lower back (lumbar or sacrum) problems are indicated. If the line is deep on the mid-tongue, problems are indicated in the area of the middle back (the thoracic spine). Deep lines toward the tip of the tongue indicate problems with the neck (the cervical spine). The tongue reflects the emotional state of a person as well as the physical. On an emotional level, a well defined center line indicates that a person tends to hold emotions or stress along the spine. When the tongue is relaxed, this line opens to an oval in shape. Becoming aware of a tendency to hold emotions and addressing it

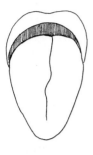

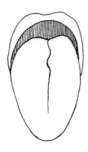

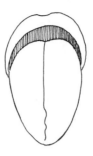

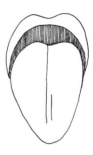

| Mid-back scoliosis | Lower back scoliosis | Shoulder/neck scoliosis | Interscapular tightness |

with massage or deep relaxation can help relieve the tightness and/or pain often associated with this condition.

If the line along the middle of the tongue is zigzag in shape, no matter where the line occurs, it may indicate scoliosis, curvature of the spine. If a zigzag curve occurs only toward the back of the tongue, scoliotic changes in the lower part of the back are indicated; a zigzag curve in the middle points to scoliotic changes in the mid-back; and a crooked line toward the front of the tongue indicates scoliotic changes in the cervical or thoracic spine. A person can have scoliosis with or without pain. Sometimes a short double line appears toward the front of the center tongue, indicating interscapular tightness.

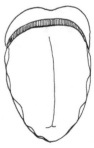

Scallops: Many people have scallops along either side of the tongue. These markings indicate problems with absorption and assimilation of minerals and may be present along with other indications of digestive problems or low digestive fire. Scallops may also indicate dehydration of the tissues.

Scalloped tongue

Geographic tongue: A tongue that is dry and cracked over the surface, called a geographic tongue, indicates chronic *vata*. This type of tongue may also be accompanied by constipation caused by dryness in the colon.

Geographic tongue

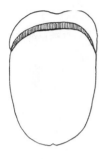

Indented
tongue

Flat or indented tip: A tongue with a flat or indented tip suggests low thyroid function, hypothyroidism. Even if lab tests indicate normal levels of the thyroid hormones (T3, T4, TSH), this marking may be present. Lab tests measure the quantity of thyroid hormones. However, they do not measure the qualitative effectiveness of the thyroid function or the presence of energetic imbalances prior to development of a diagnosable condition. If you have low energy and fatigue, the quality of your thyroid function may be involved.[15]

One thing that can be done to check the quality of your thyroid function is to take your basal temperature each morning for five days. Keep a thermometer by your bed and shake it down before you go to sleep. On awakening and with the least amount of movement possible, place the thermometer in the middle of your armpit. Stay quiet and still for at least 10 minutes and then check the temperature. Keep a record of this temperature. Your basal body temperature should be between 97.6 and 98.2 degrees Fahrenheit. Low basal body temperatures may reflect hypothyroidism, even if lab tests don't reveal thyroid dysfunction.

Stripped patches: Stripped patches on the tongue that have the appearance of a layer shaved off may indicate the presence of parasites. Excess salivation is sometimes another sign that worms are present. Excess salivation can also be a sign of diabetes.

Strawberry tongue: A tongue covered with strawberry colored dots indicates B_{12} and folic acid deficiency. This condition is particularly important to recognize and treat in pregnancy to avoid certain birth defects.

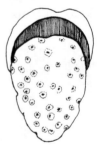

Strawberry
tongue

Canker sores: Although not usually found on the tongue, it is interesting to note that canker sores or skin eruptions in the mouth indicate high *pitta* and excessive acidity in the system. When canker sores are present, stay away from hot spicy foods and foods which create acidity, including baked goods made with refined flour and sugar. Canker sores also indicate a deficiency of B-Complex.

Location of Coatings: Now let's look at some coatings. Notice on your tongue map that the large intestine or colon is pictured at the back of the tongue near its root. The small intestine and the stomach are located in the middle area of the tongue. A thick white coating over the entire surface of the tongue indicates toxins in the entire gastrointestinal tract. However, if the white coating is located only on the back of the tongue, the toxins are confined to the colon. If the white coating is over the middle part of the tongue surface, toxins have accumulated in the small intestine and stomach. As indicated in the section on coatings, this type of white accumulation is associated with the digestive process and the power of digestive fire.

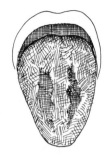

Toxins in GI tract

Locate the lung areas on the tongue map. Problems with the lungs can often be seen in these areas on either side of the tongue. A white coating represents delicate lungs. A brown color may be caused by pneumonitis. A frothy kind of damp coating indicates some problem with lung energy, perhaps congestion in the lungs or even bronchitis. Does your tongue have a coating or froth on the sides in the lung areas?

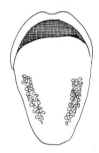

Lung froth

Notice on the tongue map that the heart is located toward the tip in the middle of the tongue. If a round depression appears in this area, consider the possibility of deepseated unresolved emotional issues, such as grief, sadness or a lack of feeling loved. A coating in the heart area indicates a delicate heart. Does your tongue have a depression or coating in the heart area?

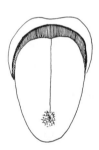

Heart imbalance

Notice the location of the kidneys on either side of the back of the tongue. If an indentation or white, yellow or even darker coatings appear in these areas, pay attention. If a coating appears along with other indications of kidney involvement as observed in the face and other areas, there could be a serious problem. See your doctor.

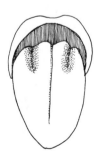

Kidney
imbalance

Putting It All Together

By now you may feel saturated with information. Let's look at three different persons, each with tongue indicators common to each constitutional type.

Vata. John is a tall lanky *vata* dominant person. He is always on the move, is nervous, has insomnia and dislikes dealing with his emotions. He thinks of himself as healthy because he jogs, works out at a gym and eats a diet that consists mostly of fruits, vegetables and salads with fat-free dressing. He has problems with gas and constipation. He thinks his worst dietary problem is his addiction to caffeine. He drinks six to eight cups of coffee a day.

John:

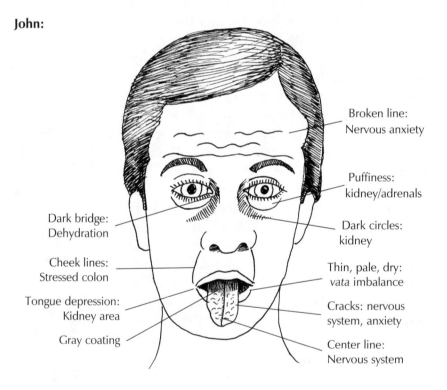

Note that the tongue and face indicate some of the same imbalances.
    Kidneys: dehydration (dryness), adrenal stress
    Colon: gas, constipation (dryness)
    Nervous system: nervousness, insomnia

Here is what we would expect to find on his tongue:
- The shape is thin, the color pale pink and the texture dry. (However, sometimes coffee makes the tongue red, because of its heat and acidity.)
- The surface has many cracks and there is a deep center line. When the tongue is relaxed and its shape becomes more oval, the center line broadens. When the tongue is tight, the line is thin and deep. This line reflects John's suppressed emotional nature.
- A depression in the kidney area of John's tongue indicates his high coffee intake, leading to stressed adrenals, which are located on top of the kidneys. The back of his tongue has a grayish coating that looks dry, reflecting the dryness of his colon, leading to problems with gas and constipation.

If you were to check John's face, you would see signs of dehydration around his eyes in the kidney areas as well as puffiness under the eyes due to stressed adrenals. His nervous nature would be reflected by the lines on his forehead. His colon problems would be indicated by the depth of the lines that extend from his nostrils to the sides of his mouth.

Pitta. Judy is a hard-driving executive in charge of a division of a Fortune 500 company. She works long hours. Her blood pressure has been rising steadily over the past three years. Judy loves hot and acidic foods and tries to include orange juice in her daily diet. For lunch, if she eats anything, it is likely to be pasta with tomato or marinara sauce and a little red meat or chicken. As much as possible, she avoids dairy and desserts.

Judy keeps a roll of Tums handy, because she has a sensitive stomach. She has much responsibility and has learned to handle difficult people well, but the effort does take a toll on her because she often must swallow her anger. Her shoulders are always tense and hard, and she loves getting a massage whenever possible. Her work schedule is erratic and that makes her eating erratic, although she tries to be conscious about her eating habits. Judy often fluctuates between constipation and diarrhea but that seems normal to her. Except for the rise in her blood pressure and the sensitivity of her stomach, Judy thinks she is healthy.

Judy's tongue reflects a variety of imbalances:
- The color of her tongue is red, the size is medium and the texture moist but not slimy. This is a typical *pitta* tongue.

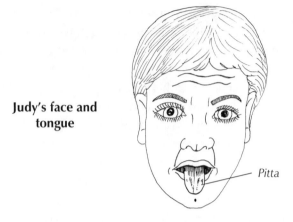

Judy's face and tongue

Pitta

- Her tongue's coating, especially at the back in the colon area, is yellowish due to her erratic colon. There is also a yellowish texture on both sides of her center line, indicating excess *pitta* in the gastrointestinal tract.
- The line down the center of her tongue is deepest toward the tip, indicating the shoulder area is where she holds her tension and sense of responsibility.
- There are several depressions in the areas for liver, spleen and heart. The liver and spleen depressions connect with her suppressed anger, and the heart depression with her high blood pressure. A stomach indentation, along with its yellowish coating, shows the sensitive nature of her digestion and her misuse of hot and acidic foods.

If you were to look at Judy's face, you would see deep lower and middle forehead lines, indicating her strong, practical nature. There are vertical liver and spleen lines. Her nose is beginning to change shape and have a slight reddish cast to it, indicating the early stages of some form of heart imbalance. There are lines from her nostrils to the sides of her mouth, reflecting her sensitive colon and stomach. Judy has a slight dimple in her chin, an indicator of the high level of frustration she often feels in performing her job.

Kapha. Carl thinks of himself as an easy-going guy who just does his job and goes home to enjoy his family. As long as he can provide well for his family, Carl is not overly eager to move up the ladder. He would much rather focus on enjoying his work and his coworkers. At home Carl and his wife like to entertain their friends and are especially fond of preparing extraordinary Italian and French cuisine on the weekends. They are also well known for their scrumptious desserts. During the week, Carl and his wife eat lightly during the day when they are each at work. Carl usually has fast food. Dinner is the big meal of the day— meat, potatoes, rice or pasta, bread, veggies and a salad. Carl's favorite foods are the sauces (especially cheese sauces), the gravies they always prepare and, of course, dessert.

After dinner Carl likes nothing better than to watch a little TV or read a bit. His health problems seem minimal. He's gained considerable weight over the last four to five years and now vows to cut back on desserts. Mostly he gets congestion in his sinuses and lungs and has sinus headaches. He feels bloated sometimes, a condition he attributes to a good meal. His fingers are often swollen, especially in the mornings.

- Carl's tongue is large, quite moist and full with a thick white coating reflecting mucus in his system. The coating is not confined to the colon or gastrointestinal tract. There are indentations and froth in the lung area reflecting his tendency to develop lung congestion.
- Carl's face looks puffy and the sides of his nose have deep indentations. Like most *kaphas* his face is fairly smooth, but with the amount of congestion and fat in his system, he is a likely candidate for heart disease and lung problems.

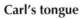

Carl's tongue

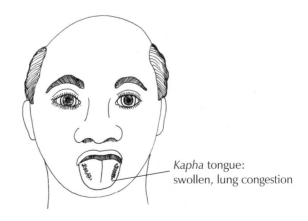

Kapha tongue: swollen, lung congestion

Care of the Tongue

It is important to know that the tongue, like the teeth, needs to be cleaned each day. Cleaning the tongue each morning with a tongue scraper is essential in order to remove accumulated toxins. Failing to clean the tongue is equal to not washing the face. Use a stainless steel tongue scraper or a spoon. With several strokes scrape the entire surface. This action will remove bacteria as well as stimulate gastric fire and digestive enzymes. It also improves one's sense of taste.

Individual Tongue Analysis			
Characteristic	**Quality**		
	Vata	*Pitta*	*Kapha*
What is the shape of your tongue?	Thin	Medium	Thick and Wide

What is the color of the tongue body?
  Healthy
  Imbalanced
	Pink
	Pale
	Blue/purple
		Pink
		Red
			Pink
			White

What is the color of the coating?	Grayish Brownish Dark brown and black: serious conditions which require medical help	Yellow	White

Is the coating thick or thin?
  Healthy
  Imbalanced
	Thin transparent coating
	Thick white coating, indicating toxins		

What is the texture?	Dry	Moist	Wet
Is the tongue swollen, trembling, stiff?	Trembling Stiff	Stiff	Swollen
Do you have a center line?	Yes (stress, tension) No (relaxed)		

Characteristic	Quality
Is the deepest part near the front, middle or back of the tongue?	Suggests points of tension along the spine
Does the center line curve?	Suggests possible scoliosis
When your tongue is relaxed, does the center line flatten to form an oval shape?	Suggests emotional nature and possible tendency to suppress emotions
Do you have canker sores?	Suggests Vitamin B complex deficiency, especially depleted B6; high *pitta* (acidity)
Do you have red dots on your tongue?	Suggests B12 and folic acid deficiency or parasites
Do you have scallops and indentations?	Suggests problems with assimilation of minerals
Do you have froth on the sides of the tongue in the lung area?	Suggests imbalance in lung energy
Are there any depressions? If so, where?	Stomach? Heart? Kidneys? Lungs? A depression suggests an imbalance in one or more *doshas* in the related organ.
Do you have any shaved patches?	Suggests parasites. Most common when a person has pets, especially dogs.

CHAPTER **4**

A "HANDS ON" LOOK AT FINGERS, NAILS AND PALMS

As WITH ALL OTHER AREAS OF THE BODY, the hand is viewed as a manifestation of consciousness. How we use our life force energy is reflected in the ways we think, the ways we conduct our lives and in the ways our bodies grow. As we change, our bodies change and our markings change accordingly.

Our basic structure changes very little but how that structure fills out gives rise to almost infinite variety. In terms of our bodies, the basic structure is determined by the shape and size of the skeletal system. That structure dictates the length and width of such parts of our bodies as our fingers and palms. Finger and palm size change very little, but individual markings on them change to reflect our personal growth and the kinds of issues we are facing.

In this chapter you will learn:
• **How to analyze your personality characteristics by the qualities that exist on your fingers and palms.**
• **How to observe and interpret major health indicators on your palm, as seen through various breaks, islands and other shapes.**

At the end of this chapter there will be a chart to help you analyze your personal and health characteristics based on the above information.

Hand analysis is not only a useful diagnostic tool but is also a great deal of fun. From the hand, you can "pick up" all kinds of interesting information about your personality as well as your state of health. Just as other parts of your body give many indications about what is happening to you, the hands also provide information. Remember that any particular indication is just that, an indication. It is not a pattern, but merely a suggestion. The more locations that contain indicators, the more severe an imbalance.

Our primary aim in hand analysis is to learn the indicators that are helpful in ascertaining the state of your health balances or imbalances. Our secondary aim is to learn the indicators that show personality characteristics. More than any other area, the hand reflects one's personality characteristics, one's uniqueness, as well as one's general health. There is almost always a relationship between our general orientation in life and the kinds of problems we encounter with our health and in our general living. For example, a person's hand might indicate that he/she is averse to risk. If that person picks a job that involves high risk, such as the job of a stockmarket day trader, the stress would predictably become overwhelming. We could be almost certain of the development of digestive problems, anxiety, insomnia, weight gain, ulcers, etc., depending on which *dosha* goes out of balance. Similarly a person who has strong intellectual curiosity, even in the absence of a formal education, will have great difficulty adjusting to a job that is dull and routine, void of intellectual challenge.

In our personal lives, those who have the trait of independence require personal relationships that give them space. If a partner is chosen who wants a great deal of attention and togetherness, the independent person will feel stiffled. This will lead to relationship problems.

We all have a tendency to kid ourselves about who we are, ranging from wanting to see ourselves as all-important, wonderful, loving, powerful, etc., to thinking we are the cause of many problems, due to lack of self-esteem. Hand markings can serve as an aid in obtaining a realistic view of who we really are.

The indicators related to personality characteristics are generally easier to observe than the markings for health, so we will start with them, looking for patterns that provide helpful information about our general psychological orientation. Then we will move on to study health issues through (1) physical observation of the hand and (2) the

major palm markings. In addition, we will learn to examine the hand for
sensitive areas and relate those areas to tissues and organs.[1]

Finger Clues to Your Personality

In examining your fingers and palms, there are several characteristics to be studied over and over—**length, width, depth, space, curvature**. Imagine building a house. The strength of any foundation is
determined by the relationship between its length, width, depth and the
space encompassed between the lines. Short, narrow, shallow walls will
support only a small structure. Large, long, wide, deep walls will
support a stronger, larger structure. Lines in your palm are similar in
function to walls. The longer and wider they are, the stronger the
"foundation," one's constitution. The more space between the lines, the
more physical and emotional space a person needs. A straight line is
linear and reflects linear approaches to life, which leave little to the
imagination. A curved line reflects elements of mystery. Think about
driving along a straight freeway. The linear straight road holds no
interest and no surprises, and we may easily find ourselves fighting to
stay alert and awake. Curved freeways with mounds hold our interest
more as we wonder what is around the corner, what awaits us, and this
helps us stay more alert.

In short, the length, width and depth of any line emphasizes the
quality of that line. The straightness of any line reflects logical, less
emotional qualities, while curvature of a line reflects intuitive, emotional qualities.

One final shape to take into consideration is **round.** There are
rounded shapes on the knuckles that indicate the intellectual orientation
of an individual. Smooth, straight knuckles indicate an intuitive orientation. Rounded spots on various parts of the hands all have meanings.
We will only present a few rounded markings, because many of the lines
associated with roundedness are quite difficult to see.

The smoothness or knobbiness of the fingers, especially the joints,
is also significant. Smooth fingers suggest an intuitive nature. Those
with knuckles and joints that are large reflect a more intellectual
approach. Additionally, the general straightness or curve of each finger

is important. The straighter the finger, the greater a person's self-confidence. When a finger is curved, self-esteem issues are a problem. The fingers and thumb usually have three divisions called phalanges. The one closest to the palm is the first phalange, the middle is the second and the distal is the third.

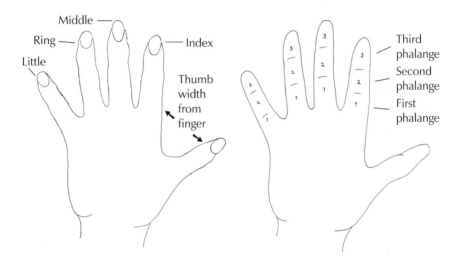

The Index Finger is related to one's level of self-esteem. Finger length, width and curvature are all significant. The longer the finger, the higher the self-esteem. A long finger is measured by looking at its length compared to the middle finger third phalange. If the length is 2/3 or more, the finger is long. If it is 1/2, the finger is medium. And if 1/3, it is short. The width of the finger is an indication of a person's leadership abilities (wide) or shyness (narrow). The width from the thumb

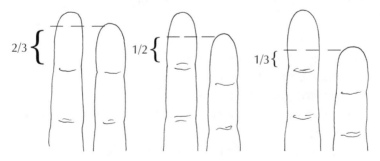

Long index finger   Medium index finger   Short index finger

indicates a person's assertiveness. Assertiveness is based, in part, on maintaining a certain emotional distance from others in order to assert what one wants done. The wider the space, the greater the assertiveness. A short, narrow index finger denotes a lack of self-esteem. This is even more the case if the finger is bent toward the middle finger. A straight index finger reflects high self-esteem and a curved one low self-esteem. When the index finger is long, wide and straight, self-esteem is far greater than when only one or two of these characteristics are present. Similarly, if the index finger is short, narrow and curved, a person clearly has significant self-esteem issues which are often masked over by compensating behaviors such as aggressiveness (as in bulliness) or arrogance.

Let's look at some examples.

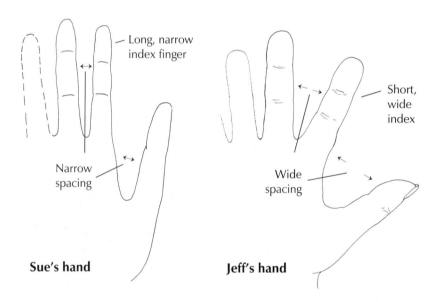

Sue's hand   Jeff's hand

Sue has long, narrow index fingers that are held closely to the thumb and middle finger. The finger length is about two-thirds of the length of the third phalange of the middle finger. Sue has good self-esteem but shies away from leadership positions or assertiveness for fear of being too aggressive.

In contrast, Jeff has a short finger that only comes up as high as the third phalange joint but the finger is wide and the space between the finger and the thumb and middle finger is quite large. Jeff has many self-esteem issues for which he tries to compensate by being aggressive and attempting to assert leadership. Efforts to be seen as a leader are viewed by his employees as bossiness, and his assertiveness is viewed as pushiness.

Now take a moment to begin observing your own hand. First, lay your hand flat on a surface with your palm down. Take a careful look at each part starting with the fingers. How long or short is your first finger, the index finger? Does it come below the third joint, the third phalange, of the middle finger next to it? Does it come up higher to about halfway up the third phalange? Higher than that, perhaps two-thirds of the way up the phalange? Is the finger wide or thin? Do the joints or knuckles stick out? How far is the index finger from the thumb? Does it stick way out or is it right up against the middle finger or somewhere in between? Is the index finger straight or bent?

The Middle Finger indicates one's level of seriousness toward life and is said to reflect business talent, reliability and steadfastness. A short finger indicates an unreliable or unsteady nature, a person who can enjoy being frivolous. The longer the finger, the more serious the person. Those with long and wide fingers tend to be good at business. Remember that width is a sign of strength, of both basic constitution and personality type.

Mark has always been in business for himself even though his middle finger is short and narrow. Though owning his own business, Mark has never been successful. He works sporadically, is poor at follow-up, is constantly behind on his bills and rarely has enough money to live on. Mark has talent and is charming so people gravitate to him, but his poor record of on-time delivery of his product and his sporadic lifestyle have precluded business success.

Mark's friend, Jane, has a long and wide middle finger. Jane is quite changeable and likes to start jobs or companies from scratch. She is a true entrepreneur and is now creating her fourth business. Jane has incredible focus though she is not particularly creative. Everything Jane touches turns into a business success, and she always rises quickly to the top of her field.

The Ring Finger. The ring finger is associated with creativity and artistry. A wide finger suggests a practical orientation, particularly when the person also has a long middle finger. Such a person might work in the research and development department of a corporation or be a graphic artist or designer. The length of the ring finger reflects the degree of risk a person is willing to take in his/her ventures. A long finger, a high risk taker; a short finger, a low risk taker. Remember that "long" means at least two-thirds the length of the third phalange of the middle finger.

Sally has a long first finger and a long ring finger. They are both more than two-thirds the length of the third phalange of the middle finger. Some of her finger joints, the ones on the index and middle fingers, are knotty. The ones on the ring and little finger are smooth. Her fingers separate when she places her hand on a table, but they separate evenly, except for the little finger that separates more. All her fingers are wide. Sally is a researcher for a high risk computer company. She works in the research and development program for new products. She is both intuitive and intellectual with great creativity along with good business sense. She is unafraid of risk but assesses it carefully. Sally is self-assured with genuine confidence in her abilities.

Frank has smooth, thin and narrow fingers with no knotty joints. His ring finger is short. He too is creative, intelligent and intuitive though not particularly oriented toward business. He works best when left alone to create and, while creative, does not want to take too many personal risks. He works as a graphics designer for a card company.

The Little Finger. The little finger is associated with both communication and sex. A long finger suggests the ability to communicate in speech and in writing, intimately with loved ones or less intimately with the public. The distance of the finger from the ring finger suggests the degree of sought for independence. If there is a large space, independence is key; with a small space, intimacy is more important. In addition, a person with a low set little finger, one that is attached to the palm a great deal lower than the other fingers, has experienced childhood difficulty with at least one parent and the emotional issues remain unresolved.

Joan and Ken came to see Shoshana as a couple. They both had long little fingers. Joan had a low-set little finger as well. On one hand each had a large separation of the little finger and ring finger. On the other hand, there was little distance. Shoshana said, "You both have issues around intimacy and independence. When you have intimacy you soon find yourself desiring personal space. And when you have lots of independence, you each crave intimacy. I just hope you have the same cycle!" Joan and Ken could hardly believe what they were hearing. They had been married for over 10 years and their respective needs for alternating periods of intimacy and independence had become the major issue of their marriage. They divorced but continued to love one another deeply. For nine years they checked on one another, and when they both were in the intimacy cycle they spent time together. This worked quite well for them. While the focus of our discussion was on intimacy and independence, Joan acknowledged that her childhood was difficult, and she still had unresolved issues with her parents.

Now turn your attention to your own hand. Examine your other fingers as you did the index finger. Look at the second finger. Check its length, width, joint size, knuckle size. Is it bent toward the index finger or ring finger? Then look at your ring finger. Is it longer or shorter than your first finger, the index finger? Is it as long as the middle finger? Check its length, width, joint and knuckle size. Does it bend toward the middle finger? Lastly, check the little finger. Does it come to the bottom of the third phalange? Does it go above the joint? Check its length, width, joint and knuckle size. Is it bent toward the ring finger?

The Thumb. The thumb shows the degree of strength of character and willpower. A long and wide thumb is often the hand of an executive, because a person with such a thumb has enough character to lead and the willpower to succeed. This is especially true when combined with long, wide first and middle fingers. The distance of the thumb from the first finger is also important. A big space, a large angle as it were, along with a long wide thumb, indicates strength of personality, intelligence, and the ability to make subtle distinctions. Thumb length denotes a person's willingness to push for what he/she wants. Width indicates strength of willpower. The second phalange indicates capacity to act and the first capacity to plan. When the bottom portion of the thumb is thinner than the top, an individual is usually sensitive and diplomatic. If very thin, he/she may not even speak up.

Thumb drawings

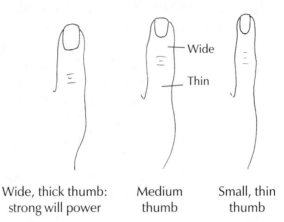

| Wide, thick thumb: strong will power | Medium thumb | Small, thin thumb |

The differences in thumb sizes below indicates that these two people could have trouble in their relationship unless one is content to be subservient.

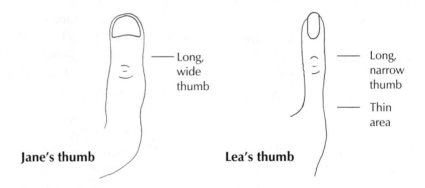

Jane's thumb   **Lea's thumb**

Jane and Lea decided to become business partners. Like most people, they did not check out their thumbs or hands to see if they were compatible. Jane has a long thumb that is wide and the first and second phalanges are about the same size. The thumb when held in a relaxed position forms a wide angle to the index finger. The second phalange is slightly smaller than the first. Lea in contrast has a long thumb that is quite thin, a short, narrow, wasted looking second phalange, a larger first phalange, which is also narrow. In a relaxed position, it is about 30 degrees from the index finger.

Right away there were difficulties in the business relationship. Jane was assertive and able to take the lead, a person who was an excellent planner with the ability and willpower to initiate her plans. She wanted a partner who could share the load equally. Lea in contrast was intimidated by Jane. While quite bright, she did not see herself as a leader and did not take the initiative when needed, and yet resented Jane doing so. When Lea felt she was about to be overwhelmed, she suppressed her emotions and withdrew. Jane tried to approach Lea gently and sensitively to discuss their differences but Lea was threatened and unresponsive to Jane's overtures. The partnership lasted less than three months. Jane took over the business.

Study your thumb. Check its length, width and distance from the index finger. Does it stick way out or is it close to the index finger? Is it straight or curved? Thick or thin? In view of these observations, what interpretations can you make about your own tendencies and personality?

Fingertips. Chances are you have not made it a practice to study either your own fingertips or those of anyone else. The principles of long and short, wide and narrow also apply here. The longer and wider, the stronger the given quality; the shorter and narrower, the weaker the quality. There are four general fingertip shapes: square, conical, pointed and spatulated. They look like the diagrams below:

Finger shapes

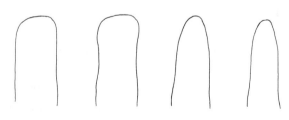

Square finger: conservative, methodical	Spatulated finger: inventive, energetic, physical	Conical finger: intuitive, analytical	Pointed finger: metaphysical

A square tip indicates a conservative, methodical person. Conservative, methodical accountants and bureaucrats come to mind as do routine and driven manual workers, all of whom are well organized. A conical tip, a rounded tip, indicates a person who can be both intuitive and analytical. A spatulated tip denotes a love of the outdoors and physical activity and an energetic, inventive mind. A pointed tip reflects an interest in the spiritual or metaphysical and inspirational matters in general. Many people have several of these patterns on different fingers.

The particular shape of a fingertip will link to the qualities of the finger. For example, a person might have a conical index and little finger, and square tipped middle and ring fingers. The index finger represents the person's self-esteem, the middle finger his/her seriousness and business acumen, the ring finger shows the creative/artistic side, and the little finger reflects relationships. We would expect, then, that this person might be quite intuitive yet practical about his/her issues regarding self-esteem and relationships (conical tips) but far more conservative and analytical about such things as business and art (square tips).

May is a self-confident businesswoman who appreciates art and values important friendships in her life. Her index, ring, and little fingers are conical, and the middle finger is square. May loves to purchase art but recognizes that she is not particularly creative herself. While she has been successful in business, her business ventures have been in unimaginative fields. She worked near the cutting edge of technology, Silicon Valley, but took positions in personnel and manufacturing for corporations that were not high-tech and whose product lines had a long life.

Finger Spacing refers to the gaps between the fingers. The wider the space between fingers when they are spread apart, the more open, independent and non-conformist the individual. The more narrow the space, the closer the fingers are to one another, the more restrained and conforming the nature of the individual. The gap between the first and second fingers reflects the degree of decision making skill, or at least willingness to make decisions even if they are not sound. The gap between the middle and ring fingers indicates the degree of independent thinking. The gap between the ring and little fingers reflects the degree of independent and unconventional approaches to relationships.

Close spacing   Medium spacing   Wide spacing

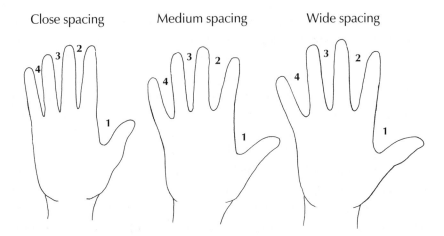

Degree of   *1. leadership*
           2. willingness to make decisions
           3. independent thinking
           4. personal desired independence
The wider the gap, the greater the quality

Fingernails. The basic nail shapes are long and narrow, wide and square, and fanned. Long, narrow fingernails are desired by many women for their inherent beauty. Little is it recognized that a long, narrow fingernail is an indication of a frail constitution. The person may be quite compassionate but will tend to have low energy.

In our society a wide fingernail is associated with men. It denotes high energy and a linear, analytical mind. A square shape, which usually also goes with width, symbolizes strength and a methodical organized nature. A fan nail suggests a sensitive nervous system. A person with

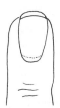   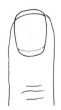   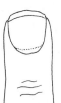

Long, narrow nail: **Wide, rounded nail:**   **Spatulated nail:**
ambitious,   strong, methodical,   sensitive nervous
materialistic,   good natured, good   system, moody, prone
delicate lungs   energy flow   to long-term illness

such a nail may deny being nervous but will be quite fidgety, constantly using fingers or hands in nervous gestures. Such a person may also have a susceptibility to joint and spinal difficulties.

Lea, who was mentioned earlier, has long fingers with conical tips and long, narrow fingernails with rounded tips. People tell her how beautiful her nails are. However, her nail shapes suggest health problems and, indeed, Lea does not have good stamina and has to be concerned about every little "bug" that comes along.

Jon, in contrast, has fan fingernails and spatulated fingers. Jon finds it difficult to be still. He is intellectual, loves to exercise and is especially fond of running. Even when he sits quietly to watch TV or read, his hands are constantly moving, rubbing against some part of his body. He is a nervous individual.

Look at your nails. Which of the shapes most nearly matches yours? Now study your hand. Place it flat or hold it straight in front of you. What are the shapes of your fingertips? Your thumb tips? Are they rounded, square, pointed, or conical (like a rounded ice cream cone)? Are they all the same? How many joints do you have on each finger? Most people have two, creating three phalanges. But some only have one and others have three. Again, look at your finger lengths.

Palm Lines: An Aid in Understanding Your Heart, Your Head and Your Life

Most people have three lines that spread across the palm. Some have only two. The top line that extends from your little finger to your index or middle finger is called the **Heart Line.** The middle line that extends from the outside of your index (first) finger, the radial side, across your palm is the **Head Line.** These two can be combined into one line called the **Simean Line.** The bottom line that curves around the thumb area is the **Life Line.**

The Heart Line. The Heart Line reflects what is happening to one's heartfelt emotions. A curved Heart Line indicates an emotional, warm person, especially when the line curves up under the index finger (the first finger). The longer the line, the more caring the person. A long line that extends almost to the outer side, the thumb side or radial side, of the index finger is said to belong to an idealistic person who is prone to sacrifice oneself to a much greater cause without experiencing much interest in a personal intimate or sexual life. If the line is curved, the person is compassionate. If the line is straight, idealism is present but warmth and compassion are replaced by a more unemotional, distant approach. A long Heart Line running almost straight across the hand indicates an idealistic, altruistic and self-sacrificing person.

A line that runs to the middle of the index finger reflects a person who is interested in choosing a mate carefully, using great discrimination. A curved line represents an emotional, caring nature; a straight line, a more analytical, intellectual approach. Both will be discriminating.

A line that runs to the space between the first two fingers again shows caring and desire for partnership. A short line that ends under the middle finger denotes someone who is more concerned about gratification than a long-term relationship. With a curved line, the person is likely to be passionate, emotional and sexual. With a straight line, the person is likely to be interested in sex, if at all, without much need for passion or emotional involvement. Sexually active people with this kind of line often find it difficult to be faithful to one partner and are not choosy about their lovers.

People with either curved or straight Heart Lines are certainly capable of being loving individuals, but the style that they use to express

Heart Lines

Long Heart Line   Short Heart Line   Medium Heart Line their feelings is markedly different. For example, when falling in love, a person with a curved line is likely to be flushed with excitement and emotion, while one with a straight line is caring and considerate but not overly emotional. In addition to length and curvature, there are also branches to be considered. A Heart Line that is branched at its end indicates a person with a complicated emotional pattern.

Great differences in the shape and lengths of the Heart Line indicate difficulties in relationship. Geri and Jim are an example. Geri has a long curved heart line that extends to the middle of her index finger and is branched. She is warm, emotional and loving and fraught with contra-dictory feelings toward her husband. Her husband Jim has a short straight heart line that ends under the middle finger. He is reserved and disdains emotional involvement. The two maintain a marriage with great emotional and physical distance. They find it most difficult to relate on any heart level.

The Head Line. Like the Heart Line, the Head Line can be straight or curved, long or short. In addition, it can spread across the palm at different slopes. The length of the line reflects the complexity of thought processes. A short line indicates a person whose thinking is practical and to the point. A longer line indicates a person whose thinking is detailed, comprehensive and analytical. Such people like to be thorough and are detail oriented. Both types can be quite intelligent. The length shows the differences in complexity and detail.

The angle of the line reflects a person's interest in stimulating creative endeavors. The greater the slope, the greater the interest.

A straight line indicates clear, concentrated thinking while a curved line reflects more imaginative, experimental thinking. The slope of the line marks the degree of creativity, whether the line is long or short, straight or curved. The less the slope, meaning the more horizontal the Head Line, the more practical the person is. This is a person who likes useful ideas. The greater the slope, the more imaginative or creative the person.

Differences in Head Line length reflect the strengths of this book's authors. Shoshana has a curved Heart Line that goes to the index finger, and her Head Line reaches horizontally from the index to the midpoint of her little finger with only a slightly downward slope. Shoshana is

Head Lines

The hands below illustrate different lengths and slopes of Head Lines.
People, however, have only one headline.

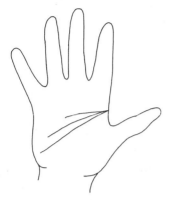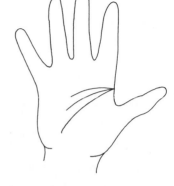

Straight lines: logical thinking   Curved lines: creativity

warm and outgoing emotionally but practical and focused intellectually. She knows what she wants to accomplish and is centered on achieving her goals. She ensured that this book stayed focused on the individual reader, and provided only information helpful to a person who wants to analyze his/her own body.

Margaret has a similar set of lines but her horizontal Head Line extends all the way to the side of her hand past her little finger. Her Heart Line is branched under her index finger, indicating complex emotions. Margaret is a compassionate and caring person who is both a comprehensive thinker and detail oriented. She loves to organize comprehensive complex material. One of her roles in writing this book was to relate the material to research and writing which reflected fresh perspectives in healthcare. She clipped numerous articles and noted studies and books supportive of the thrust of this book. In addition, she examined all the writing for internal consistency and clarity of thought and expression.

Together Shoshana and Margaret made a good team. Both are comprehensive thinkers who recognize and appreciate the strengths of the other. One look at their Heart Lines and Head Lines reflects their compatibility and differences as co-authors.

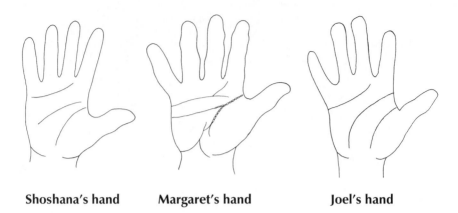

Shoshana's hand   **Margaret's hand**   **Joel's hand**

Their friend, Joel, has a different kind of hand and is a writer with a different emphasis. While his Heart Line is rather straight, his Head Line is curved and sloped. Joel is an imaginative thinker who likes to create new scenarios for how history might have been had circumstances been slightly different. He also excels in creative, imaginative poetry and science fiction. He is a creative, intelligent and imaginative writer who, in his private life, prefers to keep his emotions to himself. Indeed, his writing usually emphasizes complicated plot twists rather than the expression of heartfelt emotions.

The Life Line. The Life Line extends from the radial side of the hand, the section closest to the thumb, and extends downward around the base of the thumb with a sweep. It is often rounded like a bow. Its location with respect to the thumb indicates the strength of one's general life force. The wider the "bow" the stronger one's sense of physicality, natural energy and sense of well-being. A wide sweep but straighter line with less of a bow reflects a diminishment of those qualities. A Life Line with a narrow sweep and hence closer to the thumb suggests less vitality, lower energy and a propensity to be less happy and more ill at ease.

Sometimes the Life Line will be broken or there will be two lines running side by side. In the first case, the person will have experienced an important life change, such as a complete change of thought in how he/she wants to live. This person is likely to exert independence, breaking from family or a partner to form a new life.

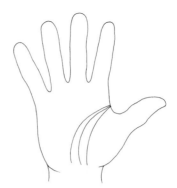

Life Line

*Any given person has one lifeline.
The illustration below shows
three lines of different distance
from the thumb.*

When there are two parallel lines, the person tends to live two different and distinctive lives. Two parallel lines can be seen, for example, in women who live "traditional" married lives inside the home while at the same time maintianing outside careers. By "traditional," we mean the appearance of subservience to the male mates while performing most of the daily household chores. While at home the focus is on the home, and career work is rarely mentioned. When away from home, the women may be dedicated to their work. They may talk very little about family with colleagues.

Lois has a narrow hand with long smooth fingers, a long Heart Line, a straight long Head Line and a narrow, broken Life Line close to the thumb. Lois loves people and has a "heart of gold." She volunteers in organizations that let her teach people to make changes that will improve their health. She is intellectual and has had two careers. For 15 years she was a scientist. More recently she changed her living circumstances, separated from her partner, moved to a new city and returned to school to study a new field, the healthcare field. Lois is not afraid of change but knows that she tires easily, can become unfocused and must rest a great deal to sustain her energy.

Rebecca, in contrast, has long knotty fingers, a curved long Heart Line, a straight Head Line, and a wide bow double Life Line with a break in the outer line. Rebecca has tried to be as traditional a homemaker as possible while simultaneously creating a career for herself outside the home. For most of her life she has lived with a domineering husband who always wants to be in control. It has taken enormous stamina to quietly separate herself from him while maintaining the marriage. Rebecca is emotionally open, intellectually astute, and has a strong constitution for which she is grateful, because she otherwise might not have the strength to stay in her marriage and maintain a career.

This section on fingers and major palm lines can provide you with many useful insights. Take each point outlined and compare it to your own hands to see which qualities are your more dominant traits. There is a chart at the end of this chapter to help you do that. Insights gained may confirm self-knowledge and/or lead to new awareness.

Your Path of Health: A Look at Special Palm Markings, Color and Nail Markings

Palm Markings. In a state of perfect health, palm lines are unbroken, deep and clear. However, almost no one has perfect health. Instead, almost everyone has lines with breaks, and even islands, stars and squares around given points. A break signifies a change, though the change may not always be related to health. A series of broken lines along a major line indicates a weakness in that line. Broken lines along the Heart Line indicate weakness in the heart energy. Broken lines along the Head Line indicate weakness in thought processes or the nervous system. Broken lines along the Life Line indicate depletion of energy leading to such things as fatigue and lack of stamina.

Common markings

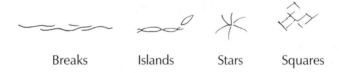

Breaks   Islands   Stars   Squares

Islands are common and their locations are significant. An island at the beginning of the heart line under the little finger indicates a history of circulatory and/or heart/stroke disease in the family at least and the development of such disease in the individual at worst. However, an island under the ring finger shows weakness in the eyes and under the middle finger an island shows weakness in the ears. At this level the nature of the weakness is not clear. Nor can we tell by islands whether problems are *vata, pitta* or *kapha* imbalances. That requires relating the markings to other symptoms. What we can gain from islands is that an imbalance of some sort is occurring or has occurred. For example, an island on the Heart Line under the ring finger suggests weakness in the eye energy. This could be a problem that calls for glasses, it could be a weak muscle, a dryness of the eyes or a tendency to develop redness or fatty tissue on the schlera, the whites of the eyes. Dry eyes are *vata*, red eyes are *pitta* and fatty yellow deposits are *kapha*. A square around a break or an island represents recovery. In the following diagrams, we will note major areas that are connected to various parts of your body. On your own hand, look for islands and broken lines. Where these exist, there is a likely imbalance of the energy supply to that associated body location.

Health Indicators

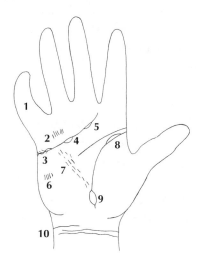

1. Reproductive organs (female)
2. Teeth
3. Heart
4. Eyes
5. Ears
6. Arthritis
7. Digestion
8. Throat/chest
9. Cancer
10. Female reproductive organs

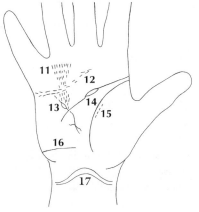

11. Kidneys
12. Broken line: Irregular heart beat
13. Lungs
14. Nerves
15. Back
16. Allergies
17. Female reproductive organs

Hand markings in the numbered areas above indicate either problems or weaknesses.[2] For example, a person with a small island in the heart area may have a propensity, perhaps genetic, to develop heart problems. With this knowledge, steps can be taken a prevent or lessen heart problems, such as adopting a diet to lower cholesterol, triglycerides and homocysteine levels, ingesting needed nutrients as supplements or herbs, getting plenty of cardiovascular exercise and learning to use relaxation techniques to lower stress. Persons with inherent energy weaknesses in any area need not suffer from associated diseases if they take preventive measures, the sooner the better. "Heart energy weakness" does not have to lead to any form of "heart disease."

Color. In addition to markings, color is important. As elsewhere on your body, the general color of hand skin is a vibrant pink, yellow, brown or black, depending on your race. Bluish tinges indicate poor circulation. Yellow color indicates liver toxins and, if spread all over the body, can signify jaundice. Yellow between the fingers and on the fingers shows either nicotine poisoning or excess Vitamin A or beta carotene. Pale white pallor indicates either nervous tension or anemia. Splotchy hands indicate malabsorption, usually from improper food combining.

Nail Markings. Nail markings change according to imbalances. In the illustration you can see the difference between a normal nail, and one that shows lung weakness with possible respiratory problems; a normal nail, and one that indicates heart trouble. There are markings that indicate mineral deficiencies, nervousness, malnutrition, delicate heart and lungs, chronic cough, chronic lung infection, chronic illness, and calcium and zinc deficiencies.

Nail markings[1]
1. Ridge: chronic illness
2. Beak: chronic cough
3. Clubbed: heart/lungs
4. Stepped or ridges: malnutrition
5. Rounded: lungs
6. White spots: mineral dificiency, usually calcium or zinc
7. Striated lines: malabsorption

Putting It All Together. Now let us examine a few hands and apply what you have learned.

Hand analysis

Conical tips: intuitive

Good self-esteem

Good business sense

Independent

Very creative

Short index

Short heart line: relatively distant emotionally

Heart line: empathetic

Eye problems

Heart imbalance

Long head line: problems in youth

Sensitive digestion

Long straight head line: comprehensive thinking

Lifeline: delicate constitution

Bowed strong life line: strong

Shawna's hand   **Mike's hand**

Shawna's hand has a long index finger that is conical with a rounded fingernail. Her ring finger is short as is her little finger, which is distant from the ring finger. Her little finger is also deeply set. Shawna's Heart Line is straight and ends under the middle finger. She has a line indicating digestive problems and an island in the eye area. Her Head Line is straight but long with a steep slope. Her Life Line has a broad sweep. Shawna's fingernails have vertical lines on all nails and little white spots on the ring finger. Her hands are slightly yellowish in color.

We can see that Shawna has a good amount of self-esteem and may indeed be a leader or manager. She has both intuitive and analytical skills (conical fingertip shape). She is not particularly creative or artistic (short ring finger). Shawna has a strong sense of independence and has probably had feelings of separation from her family since childhood (lowset little finger and wide space between little and ring finger). She probably has some difficulty communicating (short little finger) and this could mitigate against her becoming an effective leader or manager. Shawna is emotionally distant, and in her personal life has had a series of lovers that have not meant much to her. She is bright and creative in her work as a scientist, using both her strong comprehensive thinking abilities (long, straight Head Line) and her intuition (steep slope of Head Line as well as conical fingertips). However, Shawna suffers from some health problems. She notices heartburn and has sensitive diges-tion (broken lines in digestion area). She wears glasses and has light sensitivity but does not consider this a problem (island over eye area). Shawna has mineral deficiencies (vertical lines on fingernails) and calcium or zinc deficiency (white spots). She needs to reestablish balance in the kidney energy before a more serious problem occurs. Shawna does not handle emotions well and tends to suppress her anger (her hands are yellowish).

Mike has a slim hand and long fingers. The ring finger is especially long as is his little finger. He has a pointed little fingertip but square middle and ring fingertips. His Heart Line is straight and ends around the midpoint of the base of his index finger. His Head Line is long, curved and of medium slope. His Life Line is close to the thumb with very little bow. Mike has small islands at the beginning of his Heart Line and a large island at the base of his Life Line. His fingernails are slightly rounded and curve downward. There is an island on his Head Line with a box around it. Mike's hands are reddish and quite warm.

Mike is a sensitive, intelligent and intuitive person (long, smooth hands and fingers). He makes a successful living as an artist (long ring finger) whose paintings reflect metaphysical themes (pointed little finger). However, he also has a good business sense (long middle finger with square fingertips on middle and ring fingers). He is creative artistically and a decent money manager as well. Mike is a warm individual who empathizes with people easily, and who volunteers in many organizations to promote the ideals he supports (straight and long Heart Line). His creativity is also reflected in the curve, length and slope of his Head Line. Unfortunately, Mike has a delicate constitution. There is a history of circulatory, heart or stroke problems in his family, and this concerns Mike (heart islands and reddish hands). Mike exer-cises, usually jogging, to keep his heart and circulation strong. He used to be quite nervous, but jogging seems to have had a calming effect (island on Head Line with a box around it). Mike is grateful for his life and watches his diet and exercises. He practices meditation and yoga to manage the stress in his life.

Sensitive Spots on Your Hands

You have become familiar with the markings on your hands. Your hands also have sensitive spots called reflex points that respond to pressure. These spots correspond to organs in the body. They are either highly sensitive acupressure points that run along your meridians, your body's energy freeways, or they are related to nerve endings. The body, indeed, is an amazing "instrument" that you can learn to understand and "play" by learning these reflex points.

Take a minute or two to feel your hand, using enough pressure to discover any tender spots. Start with the thumb and feel up and down the sides, rub the tip, use your other thumb to exert pressure. Then examine each finger the same way, rubbing the skin between the fingers as you go along. In a circular motion, rub each pad under your fingers, again noticing any sensitive spots. Make your way down the entire palm. Do the same thing on the other side.

Now look at the chart below and you will see various reflex points. Almost all of us have had the experience of sitting on a doctor's examining table and having the doctor tap our knee to see how far it jerks, if at all. That is a reflex action. How the knee moves gives clues to the doctor about what is happening in your body. In a similar way, the body has reflex points in the hands. Notice that the areas connected to the head are in the uppermost part of your hand. Those with the lower part of your body, such as the colon and the reproductive system, are in the lower part of your hand. Now relate sensitive areas to reflex points. You may wish to write down locations. Give the sensitive areas a little TLC (tender loving care), rubbing them in a clockwise circular direction. Rubbing that way stimulates the nerve endings and sends messages along the nerves to the appropriate organs, glands, or other body parts.

One of the best things any of us can do to help take the load of stress off a sensitive body part is to regularly massage its related hand area. Most of us look at massage as an indulgence. But it has an important therapeutic function. Just rubbing your hands as described above can work wonders.

Bob developed a sore arm and the intestinal and gallbladder areas on his hands were quite sensitive, as were other major intestinal and

Hand Reflexology Chart

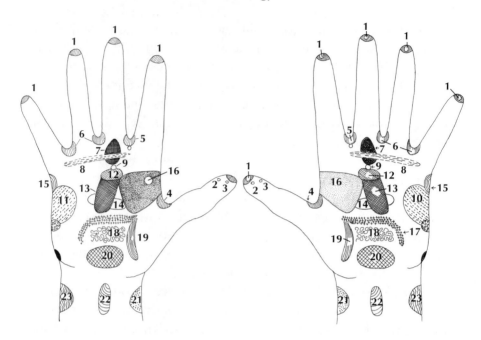

Right

  1. Sinus
  2. Pituitary
  3. Penal
  4. Parathyroid
  5. Eyes
  6. Ears
  7. Thymus
  8. Lung
  9. Solar Plexus
  10. Heart (left hand)
  11. Liver (right hand)

Left

  12. Adrenals
  13. Kidneys
  14. Pancreas
  15. Shoulder
  16. Stomach
  17. Colon
  18. Small intestines
  19. Thyroid/parathyroid
  20. Bladder
  21. Prostate, penis (male)
       Uterus (female)
  22. Lower lumbar
  23. Ovaries (female)
       Testes (male

gallbladder accupressure points on his body. Bob had pulled his biceps muscle slightly at the gym as he tried to increase weights on a machine. At first, the discomfort was only slight. A day or so after the gym incident, he went on a weekend trip and enjoyed dining out with friends. Each day his arm became worse, and he was not working out. He started paying attention, wondering if there might be a dietary connection between his sore arm and recent dietary patterns. Bob loves to drink wine and coffee occasionally but both are toxic to him. Within 30 minutes of ingesting either, Bob can check his tongue and see evidence of toxic reactions in his digestive system. Usually he drinks coffee and wine sparingly, only a cup or glass once or twice a week. But for five days he had both every day while visiting friends. Bob checked his tongue. Sure enough, the areas representing the colon and gastrointestinal tract were marked with white toxins. By the time he got back home, Bob's arm was so sore he could hardly sleep. Every arm movement caused pain.

Bob's arm got progressively weaker and more painful in the next three days. By the following weekend, Bob's bottom lip, which reflects the condition of the large intestine, developed sores and became chapped. These conditions all took place within a week of the initial injury. Since Bob by now was pretty sure there was a relationship between his diet, his lip marks and possibly his arm as well, he went on a fast, taking only liquids and light soups to cleanse the colon. In three days the intestinal accupressure points were barely sensitive, the discoloration on his lips lessened, and his arm was less sore. He returned slowly to a gentle, easy to digest, well balanced diet, and took anti-inflammatory oils and herbs to deal with any remaining inflammatory responses in his body. It took about as long for him to return to normal as it did to create the problems.

Bob's case illustrates that a physical injury can be worsened by improper diet. The major meridian that passed through the injured area of his arm was the large intestine meridian, and the introduction of known poisons to his system made the initial problem move from a mild strain to an almost incapacitating pain and the inability to use his arm for several days. Through all this there were also tender spots in Bob's hands. Prior to his injury, Bob was doing a thorough body massage daily and knew there were no preexisting sensitive areas. He was able to identify his imbalance and take action immediately using the tools presented in this book.

Summary

Of all the ancient diagnostic techniques discussed in this book, we personally find the analysis of face, hands and tongue to be particularly helpful, because they are easy to observe. The information gleaned can be readily utilized to understand personal imbalances. This is particularly true of the analysis of the hands. You can refer to them anytime without using a mirror. Remember that your hands' markings can change as quickly as your health changes.

Now that you have examined your hands in detail by sight and touch, you can use the following chart to identify what you discover about your own body. You may wish to make copies of the chart so that you can use it at other times to track your imbalances.

Your Personal Profile	
Review: General Quality of Fingers and Thumb	
Index	Level of self confidence
Middle	Seriousness of personality, degree of business talent, reliability, responsibility
Ring	Degree of creativity, artistic talent and risk-taking ability
Little	Communication skills, charisma and sexual qualities
Thumb	Strength of character and willpower

Finger Indicators: Look at each of your fingers and note their width, length and curvature, if any.

Wide, long	maximizes the quality of the fingers
Short, narrow	minimizes the quality of the fingers
Curvature	reflects insecurity about the qualities of that finger

Mark the appropriate indicators on your fingers

	Wide	*Long*	*Short*	*Narrow*	*Straight*	*Curved*
Index:						
Middle:						
Ring:						
Little:						
Thumb:						

Fingertips: Note the shape of the tip on each of your fingers and thumb

Square	conservative and methodical
Conical	both intuitive and analytical
Spatulated	inventive mind, energetic, likes outdoor activity/ exercise
Pointed	attracted to inspiration, metaphysical, spiritual matters
	May be attracted to gambling (trusts in luck)

Mark the indicators on your fingers

	Square	*Conical*	*Spatulated*	*Pointed*
Index:				
Middle:				
Ring:				
Little:				
Thumb:				

General Qualities of Nail Shapes

Long and narrow	low energy, low stamina, compassion, sensitivity
Wide	strong constitution, linear and analytical thinking, high energy
Square	strong, organized
Fan	sensitive nervous system

Mark the indicators for your nails

	Long & narrow	Wide	Square	Fan
Index:				
Middle:				
Ring:				
Little:				
Thumb:				

General Indicators for Finger Spacing

Wide	open, independent, non-conformist
Narrow	more conformist, less flexible

Gaps Between Fingers

Index & Middle	decision-making skills
Middle & Ring	independent thinking ability
Ring & Little	independent, unconventional relationships
Thumb & Index	willpower and strength

Heart Line: Check which characteristics apply to you

Length

_____ Line extends to middle finger: strong sexual nature, not choosy

_____ Line extends to index finger: compassionate, discriminating in partners

_____ Line extend to center of index finger or beyond: idealistic, prone to self-sacrifice for cause, or caring and helping others

Curvature

_____ Curved: emotional, compassionate, warm, affectionate

_____ Straight: less emotional, considerate, cool, thoughtful

Health Markings on the Heart Line

Problem Markings: Islands, broken, lines, stars
Problem areas with boxes around them: protection

_____ Heart area: on line under little finger

_____ Eyes: on line under ring finger

_____ Ears: under middle finger

_____ Teeth: above heart line between little and ring fingers

---

Head Line: Highlight or check that which applies to you

Length

_____ Long: reflects complexity of thought processes; comprehensive, analytical, detail oriented
_____ Short: practical "to the point" orientation

Curvature

_____ Curved: clear, focused, concentrated thinking

_____ Straight: imaginative, experimental, creative thinking

Health Markings on the Head Line—Problem Areas

_____ Nervous system: under middle finger

_____ Lungs: under ring finger

Life Line: Check the characteristics that apply to you

Closeness to thumb

_____ Close bow: sensitive, low vitality

_____ Wide bow: strong constitution, energetic

Shape of line

_____ Straight: diminished strength and energy

_____ Curved: enhancement of strength and energy

Health Marking on Life Line—Problem Areas

_____ Throat, chest, lungs: near radial edge, close to thumb, on line under index finger

_____ Back: on line under middle finger

_____ Cancer: island near bottom of life line

For other health conditions, note the areas where you have markings

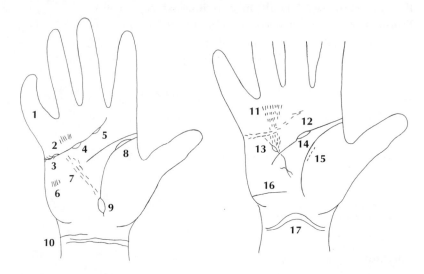

1. Reproductive organs -
   bent little finger
2. Teeth - broken lines
3. Heart - chained lines on
   heart line
4. Eyes - island near midpoint
   of heart line
5. Ears - island near far end of
   heart line
6. Arthritis - broken lines
7. Digestion - broken diagonal
   line across palm
8. Throat/chest - island near
   start of life line
9. Cancer - island near end of
   life line
10. Female reproductive
    organs - wrist line

11. Kidneys - broken lines under
    ring finger
12. Irregular heart beat -
    broken, spaced lines of
    heart line
13. Lungs - island on diagonal
    line
14. Nerves - island on head line
15. Back - line inside lifeline
16. Allergies/oxins - line near
    bottom of palm
17. Female reproductive
    organs - wrist lines

Hand Reflex Points: Put an x on all the sensitive spots on your hand and check to see what body parts are related to the sensitive areas.

Hand Reflexology Chart

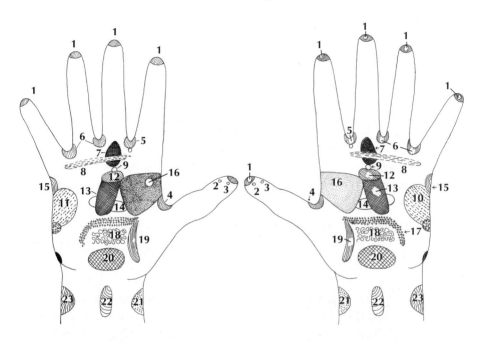

Right

1. Sinus
2. Pituitary
3. Penal
4. Parathyroid
5. Eyes
6. Ears
7. Thymus
8. Lung
9. Solar Plexus
10. Heart (left hand)
11. Liver (right hand)

Left

12. Adrenals
13. Kidneys
14. Pancreas
15. Shoulder
16. Stomach
17. Colon
18. Small intestines
19. Thyroid/parathyroid
20. Bladder
21. Prostate, penis (male)
    Uterus (female)
22. Lower lumbar
23. Ovaries (female)
    Testes (male

CHAPTER 5

CHECKING OUT THE REST OF YOU: YOUR EYES, EARS AND FEET

CAREFUL STUDY OF YOUR FACE, TONGUE AND HANDS has provided you with overlays of information about the state of your *doshas*. The more overlays observed, the more advanced the state of imbalance in that particular area. This section provides still more overlays. Once you have identified problems and energy imbalances related to particular organs or tissues, you can then compare any qualities observed in the areas to the list of characteristics or qualities associated with the *doshas*. Identifying a quality as *vata, pitta* or *kapha* gives even more information about the imbalance. For example, your observations indicate some imbalance in the lung area, and your experience is frequent congestion in the lungs—colds, flus and the like. If the qualities of the phlegm you produce include heavy, wet, slimy, smooth, dense and cool, *kapha* is indicated. If the phlegm is hot and green or yellow, *pitta* is indicated. There is a chart at the end of this chapter to help you interpret your observations and link them to the qualities of the *doshas*.

Upon completion of this chapter, you will be able to identify changes in your *doshas* by markings on your eyes, ears and feet.
Observing your EYES, you will be able to
- Identify problem areas reflected in the irises by your organs and tissues.
- Identify major markings by color and shape.
Observing your EARS, you will be able to
- Check for tendencies for high cholesterol, diabetes, and even imbalances associated with the heart.
- Identify indicators which give information about your circulation, nervous and digestive systems.

- **Identify reflex points.**

Observing your FEET, you will be able to

- **Identify sensitive spots and their relationship to your organs and systems.**
- **Relate the way you hold your feet and wear your shoes to propensities to develop particular kinds of imbalances.**

Your Eyes: A Key to Your Soul

The difficulty for a beginner in eye analysis is seeing into the eye, primarily into the iris. To "examine" your eyes with strong but not glaring lighting, a magnifying glass (if needed) and an eye chart nearby is a challenging balancing act. This is one instance where it might be helpful for you to get together with someone else. Barring this, using a specialized lighted magnifying mirror can be helpful. See Resources section in the Appendix at the end of this book.

Given the difficulty of seeing into the eye clearly, we will deal here with only its most obvious markings. In every eye there are three easily observable parts—the schlera, the iris and the pupil. The schlera is the white of the eye, the iris is the circular part that gives color to the eye, and the pupil is the black part in the center. Like the head, tongue and hands, the eyes have reflex points that connect to every part of the body. These reflex points are located in the iris, which is why we focus primarily on it.

In iridology different areas of the iris are associated with particular problems. The flow from the top of the iris, the "12 o'clock position," starts with the brain and descends on both sides, following the body's own pattern, to the legs and feet at the "6 o'clock position." We have designated these areas with drawings of the respective organs. As you use the charts, look for the kinds of markings described in this chapter in your own eyes, checking the general "clock" location and then checking proximity to the pupil or schlera.

When you look in a mirror, the eye on the right side of the mirror will correspond to your right eye. However if you are looking at another person's eye, he/she will be facing you head on and the images will be reversed. The right eye will be on your left side and the left eye will be on your right side.

Look now at the eye chart below to become familiar with organ locations.

In an eye chart that is laid out like the numbering on a clock, the numbers that are outside the circle representing the iris reveal the location of organs or various bodily systems. The top part, from approximately an 11:00 o'clock position to 1:00 o'clock, is the cerebrum, the brain area. On your left eye from 1:00 to 2:00 is the face area and from 10:00 to 11:00 the neck area. This pattern is reversed on the right eye. Between 2:00 and 3:00 on the left eye and 9:00 and 10:00 on

---

Eye analysis

Iridology Chart: *Mirror Image (If another person is observing, he/she will look into the right part of your face to observe your left eye when you are facing one another)*

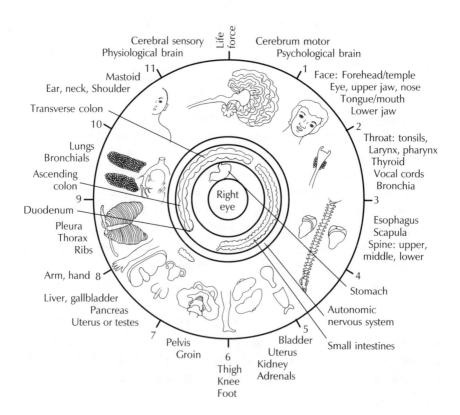

the right eye there are upper torso areas—esophagus, lungs, heart, etc. From 4:00 to 5:00 on the right and 7:00 to 8:00 on the left there are the mid-torso pleura, breasts, spleen, liver and diaphragm. The lower section of the iris, from 5:00 to 7:00 o'clock, contains the reflexes for the lower part of your torso and your extremities: kidneys, reproductive organs, pelvis, legs, knees and feet.

For our purposes, we have created a chart to show the areas that can be most readily seen.[1] Both of us have studied Ayurvedic eye analysis as well as Western eye analysis. To us it is amazing that the great Ayurvedic teachers developed this system thousands of years ago and it differs little from charts developed in Germany and the United States in this century![2]

In studying the eye, there is a natural tendency to progress from the pupil in the center outward or from the iris rim inward to the pupil. There are zones in the iris that in Ayurveda correspond to the energy

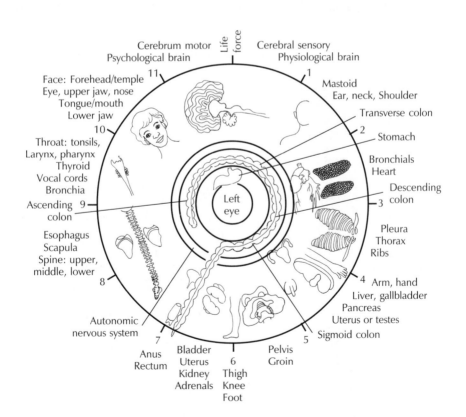

supply to the "tissues"—the skin and lymph, the circulatory system, the muscle and adipose (fat) systems, and the muscular, skeletal, nervous and reproductive systems. In the West the word "tissues" generally refers to the physical systems. However, in Ayurveda it also refers to the supply of energy to the tissues. Markings in any of these zones indicate an energy imbalance in the location of the organ or body area connected with that system. For example, a marking in the liver area in the adipose tissue zone would lead us to ask about fatty tissue in the liver, fat metabolism problems and cholesterol levels. Similarly, a marking in the lung area in the circulation "tissue" zone would bring up questions about circulation with respect to the lungs, including lung capacity, the presence or absence of mucus and breathing patterns. Are inhalations and exhalations even? Deep or shallow? We would even ask questions about the relationship of the venous artery to the lungs. For example, is the blood being properly oxygenated by the lungs?

The chart below indicates the approximate tissue areas. If you have a magnifying glass and can see the eye well, you can probably pinpoint

Tissue area analysis

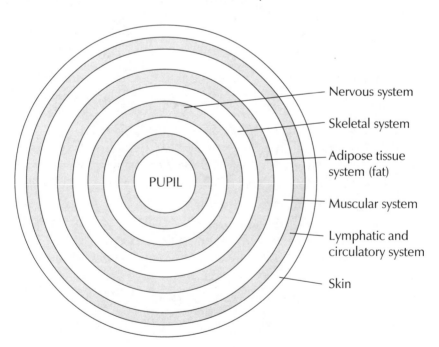

- Nervous system
- Skeletal system
- Adipose tissue system (fat)
- Muscular system
- Lymphatic and circulatory system
- Skin

PUPIL

the tissue areas. If not, just remember that the areas closest to the outside perimeter of the iris are the skin, lymph and circulation energy areas. In the middle are the muscle and adipose (fat) tissue areas. Closer to the pupil are energy supply areas of the skeletal, nervous and reproductive systems. It is important to make a distinction between nervous energy and the nervous system; between sexual energy and the reproductive organs. We always have a nervous system, but our nervous energy can be relaxed or jangled. Or we can have plenty of energy or too much (i.e., hyperactivity) or too little (i.e., fatigue). We have reproductive organs but our sexual energy comes and goes. For example, even if the organs are removed, sexual energy is still present. A woman with a hysterectomy can still experience sexual desire.

At a workshop one weekend at the Ayurvedic Institute in Albuquerque, Shoshana and an opthalmologist teamed together. She was interested in learning to use an ophthalmoscope and he was interested in learning about the markings on the eyes from an Ayurvedic perspective. One of their class members volunteered to have his eyes dilated, and they began an examination. For Shoshana it was fascinating to see the retina and internal parts of the eye. But what caught her attention was a blockage, a cloudy substance covering the colon energy area of the volunteer's iris. To the ophthalmologist the cloudy patch indicated glaucoma. To Shoshana it indicated that the volunteer had a serious colon problem. The cloudiness of glaucoma was thickest in the first two "tissue" layers, the surface layers. It penetrated through the first four layers of the "tissues." Hence they concluded that not only were there colon problems, but these problems also affected several tissue layers—the skin, lymph, muscles and adipose tissue layers. Dr. Lad confirmed the relationship between glaucoma and the colon in this particular person, and the volunteer friend was able to confirm that he had serious colon problems. This experience demonstrated that these kinds of eye markings can indeed have profound significance.

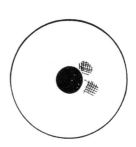

Glaucoma
clouding

Iris Colors. Regardless of the basic color and pattern of your eyes, you are likely to see little patches of pigment on the iris that are orange, rust, red, yellow, brown, white or black. Here is a brief synopsis of the significance of each:

Yellow — light and straw colored: possible kidney or bladder energy imbalances

    — dirty and pus colored: general tendency for infections of all kinds

    — ocher or dark yellow: liver/gallbladder weakness

Orange — liver and pancreas imbalance

Red — true red: kidney imbalance

    — red-yellow: liver/kidney imbalance

    — dark red: liver/pancreas imbalance (more longstanding than orange color) if located near the wreath, which is the area adjacent to the pupil. Dark red can also appear as "large" pigments in the liver/pancreas areas.

Rust — pancreas/liver imbalance generally but, if close to the pupil, colon and digestive disturbance

Rust/Brown — pancreas-blood sugar problems or problems with fluctuating energy

Brown — liver or colon imbalance[3]

White — usually a sign of an acute condition such as inflammation

Black — a sign of a developing chronic, degenerative problem

Iris Markings. There are many markings on the iris, but we will concentrate only on those most easy to observe, including markings around the iris rim and within the iris itself.[4]

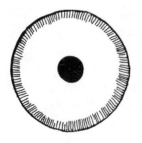

• *Scurf Rim.* The Scurf Rim is a band around the edge of the iris, either dark bluish or white in color. It indicates retention of toxins within the entire organism. A white ring indicates elevated cholesterol and consequent tendency to have hardening of the arteries.

- *Radii Solaris.* Spokes generating from the pupil outward indicate a high level of tension as well as a vulnerability to parasites. Many people have parasites without knowing it. Being free of parasites in the colon does not necessarily indicate freedom from them elsewhere in the body.

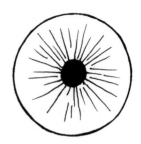

- *Lymphatic Rosary.* The look of "beads" ringing the edge of the iris indicates a tendency for lymphatic congestion.

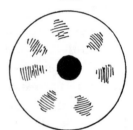

- *Uric Acid Diathesis.* In the center rings of the iris, the appearance of light cloud-type shapes indicate kidney/bladder imbalances that can lead to excess uric acid in the body.

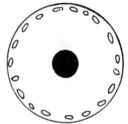

- *Nerve Rings* are rings that circle within the iris around the pupil. The rings are separated or broken in different areas. If you have a nerve ring, check the chart to see which of your body areas is affected. In our high stress society nerve rings are quite common.

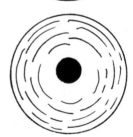

- *Lesions.* There are many different shapes to these markings. Some look like dots or honeycombs. There are oval shapes, beak shapes and squares. Regardless of their shapes, take these markings as indications of energy imbalances in the involved areas. Imbalances do not automatically lead to physical problems, especially when restorative actions are taken.

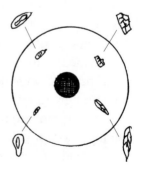

Now take a moment to check your iris to locate any special markings such as dots, broken lines, and the markings described above. Then check your chart to find the corresponding organs. Next, check the chart to observe the approximate tissue level affected. We use the seven "tissue" level chart and the organ reflex area chart together. For your purposes do not be overly concerned about the precise interpretation of a marking. Simply note the organ associated with it and the tissue energy level. You will be looking for general confirmation of observations made on the face, tongue and hands.

Both of Shoshana's grandmothers died at a young age from cancer, and since a little girl she has been aware of a cancer risk. From adulthood she has eaten few foods containing preservatives, known to be carcinogenic. She learned meditation and yoga to calm her nervous system. And later she became aware of the importance of essential fatty acids, vitamins, minerals and other nutrients. She has had three different types of pre-cancerous conditions, all of which have been reversed without the use of drugs, and she remains cancer free. In writing this book Shoshana has been able to focus on only one activity. She has been able to relax to such an extent that the nerve rings in her irises have begun to disappear. Writing has also given her the opportunity to improve her diet, that has resulted in a lightening and clearing of the scurf rim around her irises.

The Pupils

Pupil size can vary, particularly in response to light. With intense light, normal pupils shrink, and with dimness, they expand. For our purposes size is not nearly as important as changes in size. If pupils constrict regardless of light, that is usually an indication of drug involvement, often cocaine. If they expand, again there may be drug involvement, often alcohol.

If pupils change quickly, contracting and expanding in rapid cycles even though lighting remains constant, there may be too much adrenal output that can lead to adrenal exhaustion. This is easily observed after the ingestion of coffee or caffeinated soft drinks. If you drink either, take a good look in a mirror to observe this cycle. If it is present, it is a warning signal suggesting you should take better care of your adrenals.

Pupil sizes

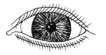 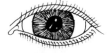 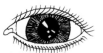

Small pupil   Medium pupil   Large pupil

General Markings and Your Digestive Tract

The major areas where people develop imbalances are in the digestive tract, from the mouth to the rectum and all points in between. In both Eastern medicine and in Western functional medicine, which involves a scientific study of the disease process, a link between problems in the digestive system and other diseases is recognized. Here in the West this relationship is only now becoming apparent as more sophisticated scanning and laboratory techniques allow us to study chemical interactions in living people. However, in the East a link has been known for some time, because the "home sites" of *vata, pitta* and *kapha* are all in the digestive tract. *Vata* is said to "reside" in the colon, and the first sign of a *vata* imbalance occurs there, usually in the form of gas or constipation. *Pitta* "resides" in the small intestines. The first sign of a *pitta* related problem occurs there, most frequently as nausea. *Kapha* "resides" in the stomach, and one of the first indications of a *kapha* imbalance is slower digestion and metabolism as a result of excess mucus and depleted hydrochloric acid. In Ayurveda it is thought that almost all disease starts in the gastrointestinal tract. Certainly imbalances of *vata, pitta* and *kapha* on the physical level all start there.

High levels of toxins ingested—through foods, chemicals, drugs, fumes, air and even toxic, negative thought patterns—all affect the GI tract. Stress is high for most people. The combination of some form of toxins and stress initially leads to energy imbalances and then to physical difficulties at the "homesite." Often what begins as a digestive energy imbalance, with increases in *vata, pitta* or *kapha,* spills over into other areas. The excess *vata, pitta,* or *kapha* then searches for a new "home" in one's weakest spot. While the face, tongue, and hands give helpful indications about imbalance locations, the eyes reflect the overlap of bodily organs, endocrine glands and "tissues." By locating iris markings and cross-referencing "tissue" rings, you can get more of an idea of the nature of imbalances.

Ears: Listen for the "Music of Your Body"

We all know ears allow us to hear, and we tune into sound almost every minute of the day. Sound and rhythm make music and it helps us get in touch with our feelings and insights. The outer ear, the part we can see, has a "music" of its own. It "sings out," it indicates what is happening within us when we know how to look at it.

The ears have markings just as the face, tongue, hands and feet do. The ones that are the easiest to see are lines that indicate heart, pancreatic and cholesterol problems. Their locations are indicated on the chart below. The heart line is in front of the ear, the pancreatic and cholesterol markings are on the earlobe.[5] While the heart indicator can be more than one line, the pancreatic indicator is just one line.

The ear spirals with three sets of ridges. The outside ridge represents the circulatory system. The color of this ridge can change readily. People who are inactive tend to have very little color along the outer ridge or rim of the ear. When cardiac exercise is intense, the ridge becomes reddish. If the ridge is always red, that is an indication of circulation problems involving excess. Little or no rim indicates a weak circulatory system; a large rim indicates a strong circulation system.

Ear analysis

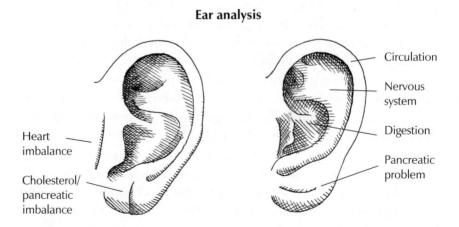

Heart imbalance

Cholesterol/ pancreatic imbalance

Circulation

Nervous system

Digestion

Pancreatic problem

The second ridge, located in the inner section of the ear, is related to the nervous system. If it is shallow and indistinct, a weak nervous system is indicated. A raised, distinct ridge indicates a strong, sensitive nervous system. The third ridge near the ear opening is related to the digestive system. A shallow ridge reflects weak digestion, a raised ridge indicates strong digestion. When there are difficulties in the above respective systems, their ear areas will become sensitive to touch. For example, if you have been eating food that is good for your constitutional type and then start eating anything you want for a few days, the digestive area of your ear may become sensitive, providing an early warning sign of digestive imbalance.[6] Rub around each ear ridge and feel for sensitve spots.

Ear reflex points

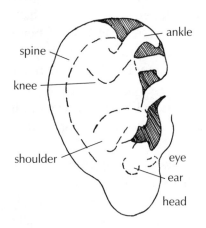

Like the hands, the ears also have reflex points. Imagine a fetus shape in the ear and note some of the key reflex points on the ear.

Your body is truly miraculous. Not only does it perform remarkably well in the face of poor lifestyle and nutrition, it also is constantly sending you messages about its state of wellness in the form of the markings you have learned about. These indicators occur long before any disease develops and, by paying attention to the indicators, you can do a great deal to reestablish balance and avoid disease. For example, the hands and ears are both quite sensitive to touch. If you make a habit of massaging them with a little oil daily, you can invigorate the nerve reflexes, sending additional energy to the pertinent organ or system, and thereby helping to release tensions before imbalances occur. Through observation and touch you can learn to read your body's signals. With these insights you can begin to make changes presented in the treatment chapters to gain more control of your health.

Foot Analysis or Why a Foot Massage Can Be So Divine!

The foot, like the hand, has reflex points related to bodily systems, and also serves as the beginning or ending point for various meridians, the body's "energy pathways." Markings on the feet provide information about imbalances just as markings on the hands and ears do.

Take a moment to treat yourself to a gentle self-massage of your hands, ears and feet. Do this before reading on. Information that is merely intellectual is interesting, but it does not help you gain control of your health. For self-massage use a little oil. If you do not have massage oil, try any cooking oil. As a last resort, use hand lotion, but it does not work as well. Use a little pressure and notice the tender spots. Locate the spots on the chart. Do they correspond to the organ, tissue or system areas you have noted on your face, tongue and hands? The feet, like the hands and ears, are sensitive to daily changes. If you eat something toxic, you will feel it the next day as a sensitive spot on your feet, as well as on your hands and ears.

Both of us, Margaret and Shoshana, like coffee, even though we recognize it isn't good for us. Margaret can drink it almost anytime with few side effects. She doesn't even get jittery. Coffee is not obviously toxic to her system. However, like all caffeine, it offers no health benefits. Shoshana, on the other hand, develops soreness in her left big toe at the liver and spleen acupressure points. If she drinks coffee once a week, this soreness is mild and causes no problems. However, if she drinks it three to four times a week, the toe becomes sore, and the toe bones start cracking when she moves her foot. If she drinks coffee every day, her whole toe becomes quite tender and her body starts to ache. So while Shoshana loves coffee, she usually drinks it only once or twice a week so that the price she pays is not too high.

Now you may ask, why would anyone eat or drink something "bad" for them when they "know" better? It is our philosophy that we

Foot Reflexology Chart

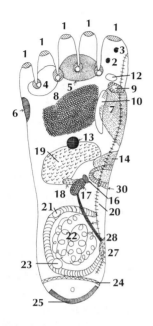 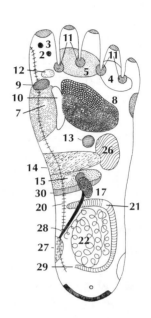

1. Sinus and teeth	11. Lymph	21. Colon
2. Pituitary	12. Neck	22. Small intestines
3. Brain	13. Solar plexus	23. Ileocecal valve/appendix
4. Chronic ear	14. Stomach	24. Sciatica nerve
5. Chronic eye	15. Pancreas	25. Pelvis
6. Shoulder	16. Adrenals	26. Spleen
7. Thyroid	17. Kidney	27. Bladder
8. Lung	18. Gallbladder	28. Ureter
9. Parathyroid	19. Liver	29. Anus
10. Esophagus, trachea, bronchi, thymus	20. Spine	30. Duodenum

do not need to strive for perfection. A rigid list of forbidden foods is a prescription for noncompliance. We ALL sometimes eat or do something we know is not good for us, and we must honestly recognize that is the case. Moderation is the key. We tell people to "pick your poisons" but pick them well with awareness of their effects on your body, and enjoy your "poisons" only occasionally. The exception to this is when a person is ill or has a life-threatening disease. Then even those little "treats" can carry a high price tag and need to be avoided. Our entire approach to healthcare is to become aware of imbalances, learn alternative ways of dealing with them, and then start where you are to make slow and gradual change. In time changes become new habits.

Now back to the feet. When you find a sensitive area, think about what you ate or did in the previous few days, until you become aware of the linkage between the sensitivity and your diet and/or lifestyle. Meanwhile, rub any sensitive area in a clockwise direction until you feel some release.

Allison experienced sore feet in the spinal reflex area and had severe back pain. She rarely went to her office, spending most of her time miserably lying in her bed. When she did get up, she had to hang on to something for support—a stick, a counter. With great difficulty and pain she saw a chiropractor, who brought temporary relief. One day as she was paying her bill, her alignment went out in front of the chiropractor. That's when she began keeping a food log. She quickly learned she had a severe reaction to shrimp and most other seafood as well. She gave up seafood and was soon walking without support or pain. During the time of her "illness," not only did her back hurt, but touching the feet in the back reflex area also caused pain. Indeed, the feet connect to all parts of the body.

Shoe Patterns

Believe it or not, the way your shoes wear can provide clues about your health. This seems almost too startling to believe. Even the way we hold our feet has significance! Take a shoe that you have worn for some time and look for wear patterns. Is the shoe worn on the inside of the sole? Outside? The toe area? The heel? The well known Oriental shiatsu teacher Ohashi maintains it is possible to do a detailed analysis of a person's lifestyle just from his/her shoes.[7] For example, worn out toe tips indicate a person who is always in a hurry. If the front part near the first two toes, the big toe and second toe, is more worn than the rest, the stomach meridian is quite active and the person is likely to be "always" hungry, physically and symbolically. The person may be nervous and impatient about the outcome of events, fearing that desires, "appetites," will not be met. Such people have a "hunger" for life, but a propensity to rush and be impatient can make them prone to accidents. When the big toe area of the shoe is more worn than the rest, the liver energy of the person tends to be excessive. The individual is likely to be driven and goal-oriented, one who is easily angered.[8]

Lewis epitomized these characteristics in his worn shoe pattern. He was always in a rush. He threw himself into an all-consuming project about every six months. If work was not demanding enough, he created major home construction projects that required almost all of his spare time. He rushed quickly from task to task, often breathing heavily. He even walked with his head thrust forward and his body following behind. His shoe tips were worn, especially around the big toe.

In contrast to Lewis, people with worn heels may suffer from kidney imbalances, and tend to be "workaholics." Eventually their kidney imbalances lead to sluggishness and fatigue. However, this does not keep them from pushing forward, usually relying on caffeine and willpower to get them through. Backaches in the kidney area are common. Such people are fearful about having enough energy to "do everything," fearful about the future, and fearful that opportunities may pass them by. They often search for personal security but have difficulty finding it.

Patterns of shoe wear

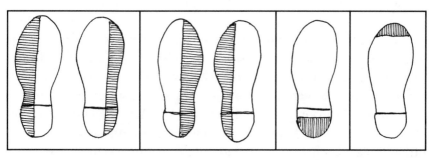

Outside worn:	*Inside worn:*	*Heel worn:*	*Tips worn:*
problems with liver or gallbladder	problem with intestine or sex organs	kidney or lower back problems	always too rushed; probably neurotic

Allison, as in the example above, not only had pain in the back of her foot but also in the kidney area. Her shoes were worn on the heel. Even while almost incapacitated, in constant pain and unable to sit upright or walk without support, she continued to compulsively push forward.

When the outside of a shoe sole is worn, the weight of the person involved is placed along the outside of the foot along the energy paths of the bladder and gallbladder. The person is likely to be bowlegged. There are likely to be imbalances in the person's bladder, and the person is likely to suffer from excess water retention and easy weight gain. Gallbladder imbalance results in increased *pitta* that leads to hostility, anger and fear, as well as physical pain in the shoulders.

The person who wears the inside of both shoe soles, especially near the arch, readily experiences liver and spleen problems, since the energy paths of those organs run along the inside of the arch. The person may be knock-kneed, even if only slightly. He/she is likely to be a little timid and frustrated, particularly sexually.[9] Cartoonists have captured this image. When they want to draw a shy person who has no sex appeal, the character may be knock-kneed, timid and nerdy looking, probably sexually attractive for very few people.[10]

Stimulating Your Body Through Massage

One of the most helpful things you can do to improve your overall condition is to massage your feet (and hands and ears, also), applying pressure, rubbing the sensitive spots gently in a clockwise direction and stimulating the kidney point near the center of the sole of your foot. Remember the kidneys are the seat of the life force in Eastern medicine, so stimulation of the kidney points (along with kidney support through diet and herbs) is helpful for fatigue. Massage from the outer to the inner, moving through all the reflex areas, the Achilles tendon, and on the outside along the kidney and bladder energy pathways. Massage as firmly and as deeply as you can without generating too much pain. Use smooth non-jerking motions. Then rotate the foot in a circular, clockwise direction. Do not be surprised if there is popping as tension is released from the foot. In a few days you will feel a difference in your feet as tender spots and crystallized blockages begin to break up and disappear.

The energy pathways in the feet and arms pass through various organs as they progress through the body. It should therefore be no surprise that what happens along the pathways affects the organs. Hence, imbalances in the liver pathway would not only make for a sore toe, but could also affect the sexual organs. Additionally, pain or sensitivity could be experienced anywhere along the meridian. When the liver energy is restored to a state of balance, the pain will disappear.

Self-Assessment Summary Sheet

By now you have examined your face, tongue, hands, eyes, ears and feet for the various markings that indicate energy imbalances of *vata, pitta* or *kapha* in your organs and "tissues." The charts below will help you summarize your observations. The qualities that are associated with any particular area help you understand whether the basic nature of the imbalance is *vata, pitta* or *kapha*. If you are not sure how your symptoms relate to qualities, turn to Chapter 8 under common problems.

Qualities of Vata, Pitta, Kapha		
Vata	*Pitta*	*Kapha*
Dry	Hot	Heavy
Light	Sharp	Slow
Cold	Light	Cool
Rough	Oily	Smooth
Mobile	Liquid	Dense
Clear	Spreading (Mobile)	Oily
	Fleshy smell	Soft
		Static

The blank charts below are for your personal use in recording your specific markings.

Personal Eye Chart

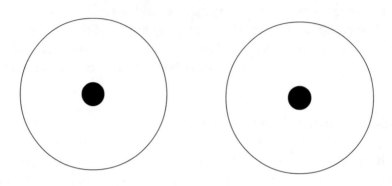

Put an X in the appropriate locations where you have markings

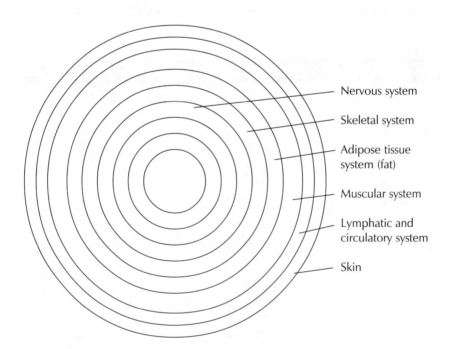

Note the areas where you have markings

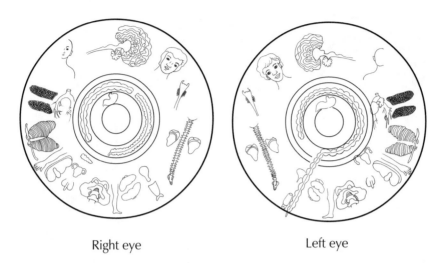

Right eye   Left eye

Personal Face Chart

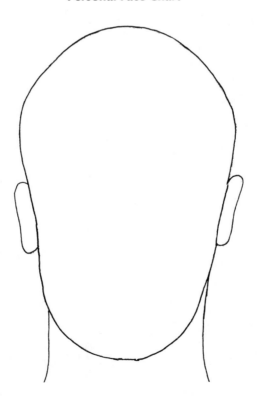

Personal Tongue Chart   **Personal Ear Chart**

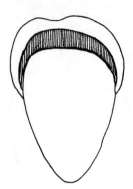 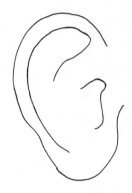 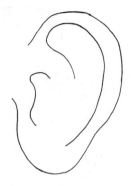

Personal Hand Chart

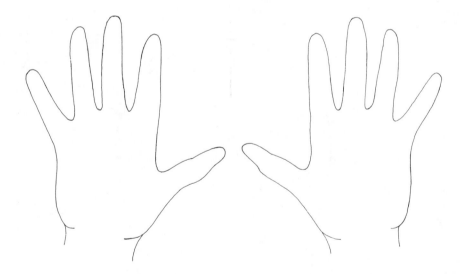

Personal Foot Chart

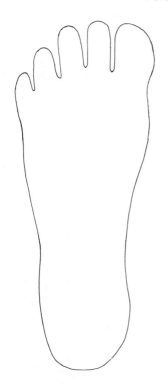
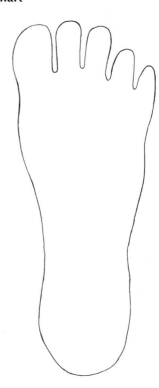

Major Organs and "Tissues"

In the chart below check the areas where you found markings.
Indicate the doshas involved.

	Face	Tongue	Hands	Eyes	Ears	Feet	Pulse	Symptoms Vata Pitta Kapha
Lungs								
Heart								
Kidney								
Bladder								
Stomach								
Small intestines								
Large intestines								
Lymph & skin								
Circulation								
Muscles								
Adipose tissue (fat)								
Skeletal								
Nervous								
Reproductive								

With this chart you have an overview of your personal imbalances and at a glance can see which are most pervasive. Use this chart with the identification of symptoms in Chapter 8. You are now ready to begin making appropriate lifestyle changes, including dietary, supplement and nutritional support. In addition, you are now ready to start exercise and relaxation programs. With patience and practice you can reestablish balance in affected areas.

CHAPTER 6

READING THE FLOW OF ENERGY IN YOUR BODY

THE LIFE FORCE IS FELT IN YOUR PULSE and is transmitted along your energy pathways, your meridians, to nerve endings all over your body.

In this chapter you will:
- **Discern the individuality of each person's pulse and how *vata, pitta* and *kapha* express energetically through the pulse.**
- **Become familiar with the main energy meridians in your body and learn to feel and observe changes along the pathways.**
- **Locate and feel the reflex points that indicate sensitivities and problem areas.**
- **Become familiar with your *chakras*, the energy centers that connect with many of your physical organs and endocrine glands.**
- **Learn of the link between the energy patterns of the *chakra* centers and physical manifestations of imbalances.**

You've Got Your Beat: Understanding Your Personal Rhythm, Your Life Force and Your Pulse

The throbbing of the pulse is the throbbing of life, the indication of the vital essence moving throughout our bodies. This throbbing life force is quite visible if you look at the top of a baby's head and observe the pulsation of the anterior fontanel (the soft spot). The tough little muscle we call the heart keeps the life force pulsing through veins and arteries, carrying oxygen and nutrients to nourish every cell.

The throb of life tells you much more than how your heart is doing its job. By feeling the pulse, a trained practitioner can determine your basic constitutional type, your current imbalances, as well as the strength or weakness of your body's organs and tissues. In the previous chapters, you learned how to look at your body and see expressions of *vata, pitta* and *kapha*. Now you can go beyond what you have already learned to *see* and experience what you can also *feel* through the pulse.

In this chapter we will show you how to feel your own pulse, as well as the pulses of family and friends, and will help you understand how each person's individuality is expressed through his/her pulse. You will learn how *vata, pitta* and *kapha* feel as the throb of the life force. The three *doshas* are a part of our total being—body, mind, consciousness— and are expressed in every aspect of our lives. The experience of feeling our *doshas* energetically is subtle, but nonetheless real.

Ayurvedic pulse assessment is complex. If you wish to study the pulse in depth, we recommend you contact the Ayurvedic Institute in Albuquerque, New Mexico. A course on pulse is offered at some time during each year. In addition, we recommend Dr. Vasant Lad's book *Secrets of the Pulse*. Although pulse assessment is best learned in a class through hands-on experience, Dr. Lad's book gives an excellent introduction to this complex art. Our purpose in this chapter is to teach you how to feel your own individuality through your pulse. We will not attempt to define balance and imbalance, as we have been able to do with the more obvious markings of the face, hands, etc., because that would involve a level of complexity beyond the scope of this book.

The pulse can be felt at many locations on the body as the movement of the life force through the arteries. Because it is convenient, accessible and gives the most complete information, the radial artery on the arm, near the thumb, is preferred for pulse assessment. Look at the illustration and find the radial artery on the inner lower arm on the side near the thumb. There is a prominent bone at the wrist. Place your index finger on the artery in your arm on the upper side of this bone. Move the tip of your finger around until you find a strong throb. Don't place your finger directly on the bone.[1] The first step is just to feel the pulse and realize it is the throbbing life force. Once you have located this throb under your index finger, vary the pressure of your finger. Experiment with how light your touch can be and still be able to feel the throb. Now intensify the pressure of your finger and feel how deep you have to go before the pulse is cut off.

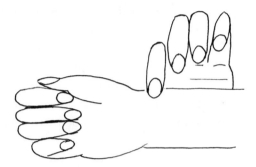

Now that you have felt the throb of the radial artery with your index finger, try the same process on the opposite arm. Some individuals have a stronger pulse on the right arm and in some the pulse is stronger on the left. Which side is stronger for you?

Finding Vata, Pitta and Kapha Pulses

Vata, pitta and *kapha* each has a special feel that can be detected through the pulse. In ancient times there were no diagnostic machines or scientific tests. Instead, early people observed nature and compared movements to those they saw in various animals. The three energies of *vata, pitta* and *kapha* were compared to the movements of a snake, a frog and a swan.

Vata has a slithery light feel, somewhat like the glide of a snake. Although *vata* is light and fluttering, it is easy to feel. The *vata* pulse moves horizontally and feels as if it is constantly changing its position. *Pitta* is a stronger throb that jumps like a frog. The force of a *pitta* pulse feels like a point coming up to hit your finger. The movement of the *pitta* pulse is vertical and is the easiest to feel and identify. *Kapha* has a deep smooth feel that can be compared to a swimming swan. A *kapha* pulse is slow and subtle, with a heavy almost dull feel. Although this pulse also moves horizontally, it is regular in feel and doesn't tend to change places as is characteristic of the *vata* pulse.

Using the tip of your index finger placed on the radial artery just above the wrist, feel the quality of your own pulse. Does it feel slithery like a snake? Does it jump like a frog? Is it gentle and gliding like a swan? This requires some imagination, but let your mind help you visualize each of these qualities. Technically each pulse type is felt at slightly different places as shown in the chart below, but for our purposes simply feel for the different qualities in the pulse.

After feeling for *vata, pitta* and *kapha* on one side, place your index finger on the radial artery of the opposite arm. Can you feel the qualities of *vata, pitta* or *kapha* on this arm? Which side is stronger?

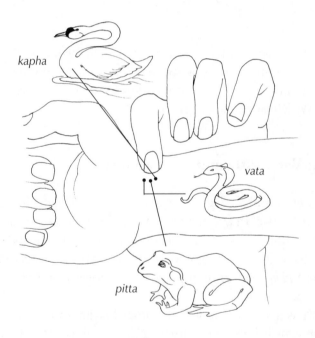

Don't expect to accomplish this exercise immediately. It will take practice. Feel the pulse of a friend. In fact, feel the pulse of anyone willing to cooperate. The more pulses you feel, the more aware you will become of the individuality of each person's vital life force. Feeling many pulses will help you determine the feel of each quality. As indicated, a *pitta* pulse is the easiest to feel. The jumping quality of the frog pulse bounds off your finger, much like a frog jumping into a pond. Determining *vata* and *kapha* pulses takes more practice.

Again, please be aware that this is subtle and difficult. We are feeling the expression of energy in the body. However, the more you practice the more aware you will become. We are all different. Become aware of these differences even on this subtle level. No two pulses feel the same, just as no two faces look the same. This flow of energy is vital to our well-being. Without it there is no life. Now let's look at some other ways in which energy expresses in our body, mind and consciousness.

Your Energy Pathways — The Meridians

Life force energy is felt as *vata, pitta* and *kapha* in the pulse. This energy is also transported throughout the body along energy pathways called meridians. The meridian pathways are familiar to many Western-ers, because acupuncture, which is based on an understanding of meridians, is now well established in the West.[2]

There are detailed charts which show the major meridians and enable you to locate them on your own body.[3] Often the aches and pains we experience as we grow older begin as nothing more than energy imbalances along the meridians. Initially they may be experienced as sensitive spots and later as pain. Generally when sensitive spots occur, there is blockage present. Massage opens up the flow, dissolving the blockage and moving stagnated energy. When energy flows freely there is no stagnation and no pain. Study of the meridians can help you link symptoms with what is happening in your body. It then becomes a task of rebalancing *vata, pitta* and *kapha*.

Do you remember being warned as a child not to run under a tree or stand in an open space or field during an electrical storm? Why? So you are not an antenna that attracts lightning. Here in the West we have little knowledge about how life force flows through our bodies. There is clearly electromagnetic energy about us. Each of us acts like an antenna for this energy. Inside the body this same energy flows along the meridians.[4] Let us now explore the pathways of the body's merid-ians. These paths are located on both sides of the body, but for simplification are shown on only one side.

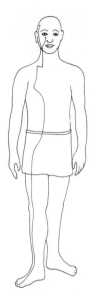

Stomach
meridian

The Stomach Meridian. The stomach meridian runs from the face to the second toe, forming a U shaped pattern on the face, then running down the neck to the sternum where it moves outwardly to the nipple area, then downward through the torso and legs to the second toe. The role of the stomach is to break down food for the small intestine. When stomach energy is depleted, there is little appetite, the legs become heavy and a person is lethargic. Psychologically, a person may feel depleted and poorly cared for by life. When stomach energy is excessive, a person may suffer from overacidity and "heartburn." Appetite can be strong, but there is a tendency to eat rapidly, without a great deal of appreciation of the food. A person with excessive stomach energy tends to have a big appetite for life, and feel ambitious yet frustrated. A chronically upset stomach reflects general dissatisfaction with life.

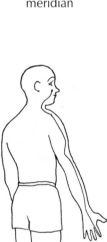

Large intestine
meridian

The Large Intestine Meridian runs from the tip of the index finger, along the outer arm, the shoulder and throat to the area outside the mouth to the side of the nostril. The large intestine eliminates waste and absorbs water and some nutrients. It has a complementary relationship with the lungs, and problems in the large intestine often affect the lungs and sinuses. Those with depleted large intestine energy may experience dryness in the colon with constipation and gas, and wetness in nasal and bronchial passages in the form of mucous congestion. When colon energy is blocked, it moves upward carrying moisture with it and settling in the lungs and sinuses. Not only does this result in problems of congestion but also bad breath. The solution to bad breath is not mouthwash but restoration of colon energy.

Psychologically, those with depleted large intestine (or gut) energy tend to be "gutless," to lack courage and determination to see their way through difficulties. Those with excess large intestine energy not only tend to have problems with congestion of the nasal and sinus passages but also tend to experience headaches, gum and tooth pain, whitish eyes, tight shoulders and/or a stiff chest. When excess energy is blocked, it moves upward instead of downward, hence problems in the lungs and sinuses. The continued presence of blocked energy leads to negativity, a general dissatisfaction with life, as if one were focused on problems and unreleased waste in life. Unblocked excess energy leads to diarrhea on the physical level. You have probably had the experience of letting go pent up emotions, feelings, etc. Do not be surprised at those times if you have a little diarrhea as well. It's just your body letting you know that release is occurring on many levels.

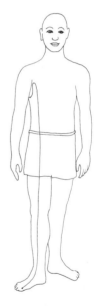

Spleen meridian

The Spleen Meridian runs from the outside of the big toe up the inside of the foot along the arch, then along the inside of the calf and knee to the torso, where it diverges to the underarm area, then turns abruptly downward for several inches. One major function of the spleen is to clean the blood of its damaged and destroyed cells. When spleen energy is weak, a person suffers from poor digestion, a lack of saliva, dry mouth, stiffness, a sensitive navel, poor circulation and susceptibility to colds. There may be an obsession with details, wakefulness at night with insomnia and mind-race, leading to chronic fatigue. Cold hands and feet are not uncommon. Too much spleen energy can create abnormal amounts of saliva, the stomach may become acidic and nervous, and there may be a strong craving for sweets.

The Heart Meridian runs from the armpit, along the inner arm and wrist to the inside of the little finger above the nail. Its function is to stimulate the heart so that blood continues to move throughout the

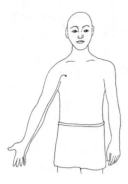

Heart meridian

system. Depleted heart energy leads to palpitations, sweaty palms, chest constriction, angina pectoris (heart pain) and heart disease. A weak heart naturally leads to fatigue, nervous tension and stress, but can also affect memory, appetite and willpower. Psychologically, the heart is associated with happiness and joy, and weak heart energy depletes both. Excessive heart energy has many of the same symptoms as depleted heart energy. However, with excessive heart energy a person may be constantly clearing the throat. Sometimes a chronic sore throat or cough is actually symptomatic of a heart condition.

A person with excess heart energy may also experience excessive thirst, stiffness, sensitive skin and shoulder and arm pain. Psychologically, such a person may be restless and in need of distraction.

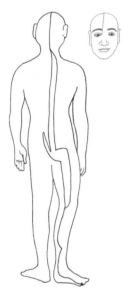

Bladder meridian

The Bladder Meridian starts from inside the corner of the eye, moves up the forehead, over the head, down the center of the back, divides into two paths at the shoulder, becomes one path again at the knees, and ends at the little toe. The function of the bladder is to collect urine for elimination. When bladder energy is weak, there may be frequent urination, incontinence and nervous tension, and poor circulation and coolness along the spine where the bladder meridian is located. Psychologically, people with bladder (and kidney) problems are fearful, sensitive and often disappointed with their life decisions. When bladder energy is excessive, there may be stiffness in the neck and migraine headaches, often the results of excessive fear.

The Small Intestine Meridian runs from the upper part of the little finger, just above the nail, travels along the outside of the arm to the triceps and shoulder blade, then up through the neck, and ends at a

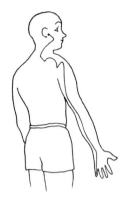

Small intestine
meridian

point directly in front of the ear. The small intestine is responsible for the assimilation of nutrients. Nutrients pass through the intestinal wall where they enter the bloodstream and are carried to every cell. The quality of our blood depends in large part on good nutrition and proper functioning of the small intestine. Diets high in fat and cholesterol coat the lining of the small intestine as well as the walls of the arteries, preventing adequate extraction of whatever nutrients are available. Cells then become undernourished and begin leaching nutrients from nearby tissues. Leaching of calcium from bones often happens, which weakens bones and teeth. Anemia and chronic fatigue also result from depleted small intestine energy. Blood stagnation in the intestines leads to complicated problems if unresolved. Headaches, lower back pain or constipation readily occur. In women, there can be PMS problems, ovarian pain or cysts. Psychologically, a person with depleted small intestine energy is likely to suffer from anxiety and to intellectualize emotions.

Excessive small intestine energy is often accompanied by neck stiffness and poor circulation in the lower extremities, cold hands and feet and fluctuation between diarrhea and constipation. Small intestine energy stays in the intestines and is not available to warm other parts of the body to help maintain both warmth and flexibility. Psychologically, those with excessive small intestine energy tend to be restless and overworked, but determined and able to finish what they begin. They also tend to withhold their emotions.[5]

The Kidney Meridian runs from the middle of the bottom of the foot, over the arch and heel, then up the inside of the leg to the sex organs, to the center of the stomach, and then to a point just below the juncture of the sternum and clavicle bones. The kidneys cleanse blood of impurities and eliminate waste through urine. In addition, in the East kidneys are said

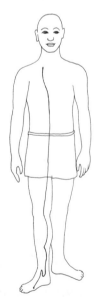

Kidney
meridian

to be the generation point, the "home," of the life force. With its pivotal role of generating and dispersing the life force, the importance of taking care of the kidneys cannot be overemphasized. The mode in the West is to ingest stimulants, especially coffee and caffeinated soft drinks, to stimulate the adrenals that lie on top of the kidneys. Look around at the popularity of coffee houses and soft drink machines and listen to how frequently people mention their exhaustion as they reach for another cup of coffee or a cola. The adrenals and kidneys are linked. Needlessly stimulating them creates problems. This is not to say that coffee and cola can never be enjoyed. The point is we need to replace fatigue with true energy manufactured by healthy bodies.

The Pericardium Meridian runs from the armpit down the inside of the arm to the middle finger. Its function is to move blood through the circulatory system. A depletion of pericardium energy leads to difficulty swallowing, susceptibility to sore throats and tonsillitis, low blood pressure and chest and rib cage pain. Psychologically, a person may become absent-minded, restless and have insomnia. Excessive pericardium energy creates high blood pressure, dizziness, stomach pain and general tightness in the hands and palms. Psychologically, a person may turn away from emotional issues, even cutting off the capacity to enjoy and express love.

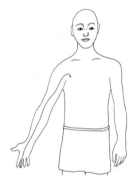

Pericardium
meridian

The Gallbladder Meridian runs from the temple around the ear and head, down the neck and along a jagged pattern on the side of the body to the hip, then along the outside of the thigh and calf to the little toe. The gallbladder produces bile that is used by the liver and small intestines to break down fats. Within the gallbladder, bile is balanced by the presence of cholesterol. If cholesterol levels become too high, the bile becomes thick, has difficulty remaining in liquid form, and gallstones are formed. With depleted gallbladder energy there is less bile, leading to poor digestion and a tendency toward diarrhea. Physically, there can be insomnia, dizziness, excess eye mucus, acid stomach and tightness in the solar plexus. Psychologically, people with low gallbladder energy tend to suppress their anger. With excess gallbladder energy many of the symptoms are the same as with depleted energy—insomnia, tightness or pain in the solar plexus, mind-race. In addition there can be a yellowish coloration in the schlera of the eye, bitterness in the mouth, shoulder pain, muscle stiffness, migraines, mucus, and cravings for sweet and sour food.[6] Psychologically, such people tend to be impatient, always in a hurry to get things done. They assume responsibility excessively.

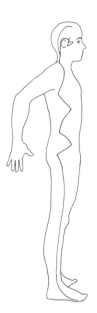

Gallbladder meridian

The Triple Heater Meridian runs from the top of the fourth finger up the arm to the shoulder, up the neck, and around the top of the ear to the temple. Those with too little Triple Heater energy tend to develop allergies, sensitive skin, tired eyes, colds, low blood pressure or headaches in the back of the head and temples. Psychologically, they tend to be obsessive. Those with too much Triple Heater energy may develop lymphatic congestion and inflammation,

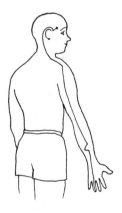

Triple heater meridian

excess mucus, poor skin tone, leg heaviness, inflammation in the gums and mouth. Psychologically, they tend to be cautious, hypersensitive and distrusting.

Although the term Triple Heater is not familiar to us in the West, this meridian is important in the East. It provides energy to the small intestine meridian and the lymphatic system and assists circulation to the extremities. This meridian also coordinates the three heating systems, which maintain the body temperature. One system is above the solar plexus, the second is in between the solar plexus and the navel, and the third is below the navel.

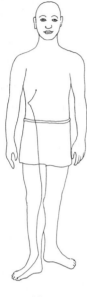

Liver
meridian

The Liver Meridian extends from the upper part of the big toe, along the top of the foot, the inner calf, thigh and pelvis, the outer abdomen to a point on the lower rib cage. Its functions are multiple—cleansing blood, storing energy, and creating immune cells and digestive enzymes. When liver energy is depleted, the liver does not release glycogen, energy from stored fuel. Initially, symptoms may only involve dizziness, fatigue, tired eyes and even a tendency to be accident prone, in part because of fatigue. However, over time more serious problems evolve, in part because of increased toxins in the liver. The problems can include lessened sexual vitality, impotence and diseases of the liver. When liver energy is excessive, a person tends to be compulsive, often becoming a workaholic or alcoholic. Because the liver meridian passes through the pelvis and reproductive organs, a pulling action along the meridian can cause tightness in the anus, hemorrhoids, prostate and testicular problems in men, and PMS and inflammation in the reproductive system in women. The accumulation of toxins may result in body odor. Psychologically, those with excess liver energy tend to be aggressive, stubborn, angry and prone to emotional outbursts.

The Lung Meridian begins from a point above the breast near the clavicle, and runs along the inside of the arm to the thumb. The lungs breathe in oxygen and the life force, and help cleanse the blood by removing carbon dioxide and infusing oxygen and the life force. Those with depleted lung energy have difficulty eliminating carbon dioxide, which then remains in the blood. They are prone to mucus, colds, viruses and tension, especially in the shoulders. Deep breathing helps eliminate tension but those with depleted lung energy do not usually practice

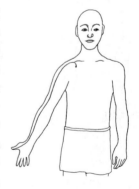

Lung meridian

deep breathing. Without sufficient oxygen they develop stagnation, easy weight gain and heaviness in the head. There can also be congestion and even a tendency toward bronchitis and asthma. Chest muscles tighten, especially along the lung meridian. Psychologically, those with low lung energy tend to become obsessive and anxious over details. They tend to experience depression, loss of memory and to have trouble releasing pent-up energy. They may feel oppressed, apprehensive and have difficulty physically expressing love.

The Chakras — Where Does Your Energy Come From?

Many ancient systems incorporate seven major energy centers called *chakras,* that are located in the same general areas as the major endocrine glands. Each energy center has a set of ideas and emotions connected with it which affect one's health.[7]

Unresolved ideas and emotions "crystallize" in the body in our weakest areas. If a *chakra* energy center contains unresolved ideas and emotions, it should be no surprise when problems develop in that area. These ideas and emotions are likely to be unconscious. We do not intentionally sit around thinking up ways to make ourselves sick. It is useless to ask ourselves how we "cause" something related to our unconscious. As we become aware of the relationship of our emotions to our physical problems, it becomes increasingly apparent that work on our emotions is as important to our health as work on the physical level.

The word *chakra* means wheel, and the swirl of energy within each *chakra* center can be visualized as a turning wheel. This swirling action is associated with the transformation of matter into energy and energy into matter, two sides of the same coin. Because of this connection, we find associations with both the emotional and physical within the *chakras*.

The First Chakra. The first *chakra* is located at the base of the torso, in the sacral plexus area, in the endocrine area of the sex organs. Physically, the first *chakra* governs the reproductive system. Emotionally it governs our sense of survival and groundedness. Dysfunctions

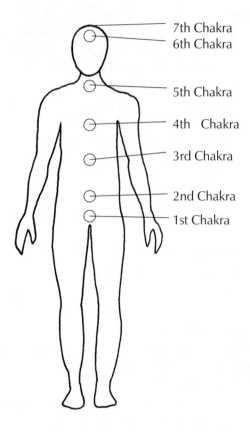

manifest as lack of groundedness and fears about survival. Those who have emotional issues about their ability to survive in the world— physically, mentally, economically and emotionally—often develop problems in the pelvic cavity. It is not uncommon for people who lose their jobs through "downsizing" to end up with back pain, particularly in the lower back, the lumbar area. Similarly those who are afraid they cannot cope with life may experience a variety of problems related to first *chakra* imbalance.

Nora was a fearful person and experienced a variety of first chakra problems. She was afraid she would become unable to support herself, partly because of health problems. Fear is a first *chakra* issue related to survival. In Nora's case, her fears manifested as numerous unresolved problems, primarily energy stagnation in the pelvic cavity, stagnation of *vata* energy, whose function it is to eliminate waste from the system (feces, urine, vaginal secretions, placenta, etc.). Nora had a hysterectomy but nothing was done to reverse the stagnation. Eventually the stagnation centered in her lower spine and she had a lumbar fusion. The back problem was relieved but the stagnation continued. From an Ayurvedic point of view, the treatment priority for Nora had to be removal of the stagnation and rebalancing of *vata*. With continued stagnation and blockage of *vata,* Nora would continue to experience one sort of pelvic problem after another.

The Second Chakra. The second *chakra* physically connects to the splenic plexus of the nervous system and to the genitourinary tract. It is functionally related to the spleen. Emotionally, its function is self-esteem and desire for procreation. Those who experience dysfunction of the second *chakra* commonly experience excessive fear and anxiety or sexual issues ranging from sexual suppression to sexual addiction. Note that the functioning of the reproductive system is located in the first *chakra,* while the desire to procreate is based on the second *chakra.* The glands related to the second *chakra* are the adrenals, and second *chakra* problems can involve the kidneys to which the adrenals are attached, as exemplified by Jason's case.

Jason was severely disappointed in his personal career decisions. Repeatedly he passed up opportunities because of low self-esteem, fear of being wrong, and of making embarrassing mistakes. He often tried to compensate by becoming arrogant and by trying to control others, especially his wife and children. He managed to get through law school but flunked the bar three times before finally passing. As a lawyer he settled for a low level government job. Jason always felt tense and stressed and generally felt both personally discontented and depressed. His adrenals were overworked by stress and excessive caffeine. Jason developed kidney problems with symptoms that initially manifested as excessive urination. Over the years he became susceptible to kidney infections and more chronic conditions.

The Third Chakra. The third *chakra,* located near the celiac plexus, is related to the pancreas and affects the digestive system. Emotionally, one's sense of personal power is associated with this *chakra*. In a dysfunctional state, there can be anger, hatred, desire for domination and excessive aggressiveness. Personal ego issues are concentrated in this *chakra*.

Ben worked for a Fortune 500 company in a sales support area and had big ego problems. As he grew older, he began to doubt his ability to keep up with his work and began to drink heavily. At the same time he became defensive about his competency. When his productivity began to slip and his superiors began to counsel with him, his reaction was to strike out against them for their inadequacies rather than to review his own performance. At the same time, he developed diabetes. Ben's emotional issues were focused on issues of competency and empowerment. His physical problems were related to his pancreas, one of the organs related to the third *chakra*.

The Fourth Chakra. The fourth *chakra* is associated with the cardiac plexus, the circulatory system, and the thymus gland. Emotionally, the *chakra* is associated with love. A common problem which accompanies a dysfunctional fourth *chakra* is to feel unloved and unlovable. Even in the West we have long associated heart energy with love and with the physical heart.

Nick was born into a family that was controlling, emotionally distant and unloving. He constantly sought approval from his parents, so much so that he selected a career based on their wishes instead of his interests. He became a counselor when he would have preferred to be an engineer. Nick did not have good interpersonal skills and never enjoyed his work. Over the years he became increasingly critical, judgmental and angry. In fact, these were the only emotions he expressed to others. Otherwise, he led a life of emotional suppression and isolation. Nick was not loving or lovable. Patterns of suppression dominated his physical as well as his emotional life. His arteries became clogged with plaque, which resulted in a lack of flow and the development of hypertension. He has already had one heart attack.

The Fifth Chakra. The fifth *chakra*, located near the cervical plexus, affects respiration and metabolism and is related to the thyroid and parathyroid glands. It is the emotional center for communication and willpower. Dysfunction can lead to communication problems ranging from withdrawn silence to compulsive talking. A person may speak freely about intellectual matters but refrain from expressing emotions. Or if verbal about emotions, a person may be unable to act on insights because of weak willpower. Others with fifth *chakra* dysfunction may have strong willpower but weak communication skills. They come across as bullies.

Janet's case demonstrates the link between fifth *chakra* dysfunction and communication. Janet has a weak thyroid, weak willpower, and good communication skills. She is intelligent, well-educated and committed to her own personal growth. However, she suffered as a child from severe abuse. As an adult she has been able to review the abuse but not to resolve the emotional damage. She recycles her painful memories so frequently that the constant recycling keeps her stuck in the past and unable to use her willpower to move ahead. Her fear manifests both psychologically and physically. Her emotional energy is stuck in her throat and she frequently has throat problems. As a nurse practitioner, Janet is aware of the relationship between her throat, her willpower, and her difficulty with communication skills. When she is particularly stuck and frustrated, her throat becomes tight and sore, and she has frequent bouts of strep throat. Unfortunately, Janet has become more and more fearful, and uses the past in a way that keeps her victimized.

The Sixth Chakra. The sixth *chakra* is related to the hypothalamus and optic chiasm. The system with which it is most closely associated is the autonomic nervous system. The associated gland is the pituitary. The sixth *chakra* is connected to intuition, and those who experience its dysfunction may be reluctant to "see" or "face" reality. They may experience a deep division between their intellectual and emotional lives. This is well demonstrated in the life of Terrance.

Terrance was extremely bright, with advanced degrees in a number of different fields. He was quietly ambitious and had several careers simultaneously, accomplishing them by working almost all the time. During his off time, he preferred to be alone, and maintained emotional distance from almost everyone, even though he interacted in his various professions with large numbers of people. Because he was charming, personable and listened well to others, many falsely believed he was a good friend. Terrance was so good at drawing others out they did not realize he was not sharing personal information about himself. Terrance

had marvelous insight and intuition, and he used these well profession-
ally. However, his approach to life emotionally was always to "mini-
mize losses" rather than to "maximize gains." He saw his cup as half
empty rather than half full, and his emotional actions were based on
preventing loss. While recognizing a capacity to love deeply, Terrance
chose to suppress his emotions and remain detached as a protection
against future emotional devastation. The price Terrance paid was
steep: there was no emotional intimacy in his life and he lived in a state
of "spiritual bankruptcy." Terrance experienced a severe imbalance in
his sixth *chakra*.

The Seventh Chakra. The seventh *chakra* is located in the cere-
bral hemisphere, and is associated with the central nervous system and
the pineal gland. Ayurvedic teachings refer to the seventh *chakra* as
the Crown Chakra, the thousand petal lotus. When it is fully opened,
a state of bliss occurs. Little has been written about the seventh
chakra, except that those who have an open one void of dysfunction
experience complete oneness with the life force. Experience of that
kind cannot be adequately described in words. People who have the
experience are able to remove any blockages of their life force flow
through awareness. By being completely honest with themselves, they
are able to view their actions, reactions and inter-relationships with
the external world as they really are—good, bad or ugly—without any
need for denial, self-deception or self-importance. This state is
achieved by those with extraordinary spiritual awareness—Jesus, Bud-
dha, Mohammed, Moses and others whom Ayurveda calls "enlight-
ened."[8]

* * * * *

The pulse, meridians and *chakras* are all expressions of the flow of
energy within our bodies. As we open ourselves to these expressions of
the life force and raise our awareness around the inter-relatedness of
matter and energy—body, mind and consciousness—we deepen our
sense of understanding of all that is, seen and unseen. This deepened
understanding is what this book is about.

The concepts of energy pathways provide the foundation for a broad range of healing practices, including Ayurvedic *marma* therapy based on acupressure points, Ayurvedic cleansing techniques called *panchakarma*, Chinese and Japanese acupuncture treatment, Western chiropractic treatment and various massage systems. Symptoms of imbalance overlap, which is part of the reason why doctors have such a difficult time diagnosing a disease process until it is well advanced with specific symptoms.

The Ayurvedic process of diagnosing energy imbalances is fascinating, and Ayurvedic treatment is straightforward. The principles are basic. If you lead an unhealthy lifestyle, you will become unhealthy. The elements that make up your lifestyle on a practical, physical level include the food you eat, your exercise pattern (or lack thereof) and how you deal with stress.

Yet it is our consciousness, the way we look at the world, that is most important. Consciousness, which is rooted in the mind through awareness, and rooted in the spirit through our spiritual beliefs about the nature of the universe and our relationship to it, determines many of our experiences, although most of us grow up thinking that our experiences determine our consciousness. We need to gain the insight that experience and consciousness each run to the other and are occurring all the time.

PART II

WHAT CAN I DO ABOUT IT?

CHAPTER 7

HOW TO IDENTIFY WHAT'S IMBALANCED: LIFESTYLE LINKS TO COMMON SYSTEM PROBLEMS

Introduction

THIS CHAPTER AND THE NEXT ONE are about treatment, but it is not treatment from a Western allopathic point of view. The approaches all focus on lifestyle changes that can have a profound effect on your health. They are not based on high-cost technology or expensive medicines. The suggested treatment modalities aim to give you a great deal of control, particularly if you are still in the early stages of the disease process with non-specific symptoms.

> **In this chapter we will discuss:**
> * **The Ayurvedic model of the disease process**
> * **The impact that food choices have on health**
> * **Steps in making successful dietary changes**
> * **Choosing proper exercise for your constitution**

Disease Doesn't Happen Overnight: The Disease Process

The concept of health is fundamental to the understanding of disease. Health is order and disease is disorder. As a pendulum which swings from side to side, the body is constantly trying to find its midpoint of balance. As stated earlier, what defines the state of balance is the relationship between the basic constitution and the current state.

When these are the same, balance is achieved. When they are not the same, the difference can be traced initially to increases in the qualities associated with the *doshas*. The state of balance, or harmony, is essential for natural resistance and immunity. *When a state of imbalance begins at any level of body, mind or consciousness, the disease process begins.*

Imbalances occur on the physical level when *vata, pitta* or *kapha*, which we call the *doshas*, become too high or too low in the body's waste systems or tissues. Waste includes urine, feces and sweat. Tissues include plasma, blood, muscle, fat, bone, nerves, bone marrow and reproductive organs. Remember that "too high" and "too low" are relative to each individual's constitution. If a person, for example, is *kapha* dominant, a K_3, then K_4 means *kapha* is too high, and K_2 means *kapha* is too low.

When we are strong and healthy, we are said to have strong immunity. In such a state of balance, our internal environment can cope with many stresses from the outer world. However, when imbalances occur and the immune system is compromised, the disease process begins.

What are some of the factors in our internal environment that create imbalance and deplete immunity? We begin with the concept of cause and effect and how violation of our own inherent common sense, our own inner wisdom, leads to initial imbalances. Initial imbalances when reinforced progress through the six levels of the disease process, which we will discuss in detail. Early symptoms are general and "nonspecific." Not until the fourth stage is a name applied and a disease diagnosis made. However, well before a disease manifests, there is a stimulus, a cause, that produces an imbalance, the effect. The *doshas* are increased or decreased through increases or decreases in one or more of the qualities associated with a given *dosha*. Imbalances then lead to disturbances of the digestive process, the "digestive fire" or metabolism. With lowered digestive fire, toxic waste builds up. When the presence of excessive qualities interferes with the digestive process, nutrients cannot be properly utilized. Undigested nutrients become waste, toxins, if not eliminated from the system. Toxins then are viewed as the basic cause of disease, because it is the spread of toxins to the tissues, organs and systems that leads to the development of symptoms that make you feel bad.

Digestive Fire. The state of the *doshas* and how they affect the body is due to the strength or weakness of our digestive fire. The concept of digestive fire involves more than just the physical digestive fire of the gastrointestinal tract. It also includes "digestion" on the mental, emotional and spiritual levels. Almost all disease involves an imbalance of digestive fire. Like all fires, the body's digestive fire changes from moment to moment. Problems can result from excess heat, primarily *pitta* conditions such as fever, inflammation and infection. Or there can be too little heat leading to malabsorption, primarily a *kapha* condition. Any action, mental or physical, that places stress on the body or mind can affect the power of digestive fire.

Harold has exceptionally strong digestive fire. His metabolism is so high that he can't put on weight. Even though he eats 3000 to 4000 calories per day, he is skinny. Harold exemplifies that hyperdigestion in the form of extremely high digestive fire can produce problems just as low digestive fire can.

Toxic Waste. When stress leads to low digestive fire, it then leads to the development of toxic waste. The concept of toxic waste includes mental, emotional and spiritual aspects of all of us. Partly digested food, thoughts or actions cannot be used by the system and tend to clog it with toxic materials which then affect immunity. These stagnant pools of undigested matter provide the environment for the breeding of disease.

Stephanie's health exemplifies low digestive fire. She loves a sedentary lifestyle and rich *kapha* provoking foods, which have the qualities of heaviness and clogging. Her sinuses are clogged, even in the summer. Sometimes she finds breathing difficult, especially at night. All year round she has sinus headaches and mucous drainage each morning. Stephanie's low digestive fire and inappropriate food choices are interrelated and are the sources of her other problems.

Because of the advent of modern drugs beginning in the late 1930s, attention has been diverted from concepts of cleansing and removal of toxins to the miracles of wonder drugs. For a while it was thought that disease could be completely eradicated by drugs. However, after over fifty years of drug therapy, it is clear that while drugs can prolong life, they are rarely a cure for disease. That awareness brings us back to the issues of cause and effect, and how disease manifests in the body. This book looks at the role of obstruction in the disease process. Where there is obstruction or blockage in the pathways of body, mind or consciousness, toxins cannot move in the normal direction of elimination, and recklessly move about the body looking for a weak place to settle. Obstruction or blockage occurs through excess accumulation of *kapha* and through decreased *pitta,* in which harmful substances are either not converted to useful substances or are not eliminated from the body. Thus the disease process begins.

The Six Stages of Disease

Each of the *doshas* has a starting point, or homebase, in the digestive tract. The "home" of *kapha* is the stomach, with its strong lining of mucous membrane. The home of *pitta* is the small intestines, where food is broken down and passed through the intestinal walls to be carried to the cells. The colon is the home of *vata,* where the body moves and eliminates waste products through excretion.

Accumulation. Ayurveda divides the development of disease into six stages. In the first stage, Accumulation, the *doshas* begin to accumulate in their respective sites. Each *dosha* produces its own characteristic symptoms. *Kapha* creates lethargy, heaviness, bloating and loss of appetite with weakened digestion. *Pitta* produces burning sensations, increased body heat, a bitter taste in the mouth, yellowness of the skin, acidity in the stomach and increased anger. *Vata* causes weakness and dryness of the body, desire for warmth, stiffness, gases, constipation, disturbed sleep, and fear and anxiety. The stage of Accumulation is the easiest to treat, because the *doshas* can be easily brought back into balance before they leave their primary locations.

The early stage of *vata, pitta* or *kapha* imbalance can be seen in a woman's response to menses. A woman who has an early *kapha* imbalance is likely to experience water retention, bloating, dull aching cramps and heavy menstrual flow. Those with an early *vata* imbalance will react quite differently, experiencing nervous tension, anxiety, insomnia and/or mood swings along with scanty flow. Women with an early imbalance of *pitta* are likely to have severe cramps, become irritable and angry, and/or experience hot spells and headaches. Their flow may be "medium," not heavy and not scanty, but it is likely to be hot or quite warm.

Aggravation. In the second stage of the disease process, Aggravation, the *doshas* continue to increase, begin to put pressure on their prime locations, and symptoms intensify. *Kapha* symptoms can include further reductions in appetite, weak digestion, nausea and excessive sleep. *Pitta* symptoms can include heartburn, belching with an acid taste, burning pain in the abdomen, loss of body strength and diminished sleep. *Vata* can develop increased constipation, pain or cramping in the abdomen, accumulation of gas and gurglings in the colon. Treatment is still relatively easy at this stage of disease development.

Overflow or Spread. If the aggravated *doshas* are allowed to proceed unchecked, they overflow their primary locations and wander about the body looking for a place to land, "weak spots." All previous symptoms worsen. In this third stage of disease, called Overflow or Spread, *kapha* can develop lack of taste in the mouth, increased salivation, nausea and vomiting. *Pitta* can develop burning diarrhea, pain during digestion of food and increase in body heat. *Vata* can create colicky pain in the colon, painful defecation with copious gas, body weakness and impairment of the motor and sensory nerves. Initially excess *doshas* overflow into the digestive system, but later are carried to other parts of the body.

Bob has a sensitive digestive system and has imbalances in two of his *doshas*. He is easily constipated, a *vata* symptom of dryness. He has acid indigestion, a *pitta* symptom of heat. When he is under any stress at all, he must restrict his food choices to bland foods, such as rice or bland chicken broth with no spices of any kind. If he doesn't do so, Bob will develop severe diarrhea until one of two things occurs: he is no longer under stress, or he moves to a restricted diet.

Deposition or Infiltration. In stage four of the disease process, Deposition or Infiltration, the early indicators of disease appear. When the circulating *doshas* find the "right" location (meaning your weakest spot) in which to concentrate, they begin to initiate a specific illness. By stopping the disease process at this stage, the body can heal itself with less danger of lasting effects. The symptoms that appear at this stage are different for each condition. For example, in early symptoms preceding tuberculosis a person experiences a rise of temperature and burning hands and feet in the evening. Preceding diabetes there is increased frequency of urination, especially at night, sweet taste in the mouth and up and down cycles of energy. Prior to arthritis there is stiffness and cracking in the joint. By the time a person arrives at this fourth stage of the disease process, it is not at all unlikely that all three *doshas—vata, pitta, kapha*—are imbalanced to some degree.

George typifies a person with multiple imbalances. He suffers from sinus and lung congestion (*kapha*), that readily lead to colds and flus and easily develop into inflammatory sinusitis in the nasal cavity and/or bronchitis in the lungs (both are *pitta*). His legs swell and he has water retention (*kapha*). George has ulcers (*pitta*). Because of his ulcer, George all too often skips meals. He eats sporadically, staying away from hot or acidic foods, but eats foods that readily produce gas and constipation (*vata*)—dry foods, broccoli, cabbage, brussels sprouts and cauliflower. All of George's *doshas* are imbalanced.

Manifestation. In the fifth stage of disease development, Manifestation, the symptoms characteristic of a disease fully manifest and diagnosis is no longer in doubt. This is the stage in which allopathic medical doctors can be quite helpful, because it is at this stage that tests point to a specific diagnosable disease or diseases. Symptoms are more specific than earlier, test results are more conclusive and treatment protocols may be explicit. However, disease at this stage is confined to a given area. Drugs or surgical intervention can be helpful. Cancer can be removed before it has spread to other tissues or organs. A pacemaker can reestablish a strong heart rhythm. Knee surgery can help compensate for missing cartilage and free a person from arthritic pain. The list of the benefits of medical intervention at this stage is extensive.

Destruction of Tissues with Complications. In the final stage of disease development, Destruction of Tissues with Complications, disease has completely manifested, has spread to other tissues, organs or systems, and is quite difficult or impossible to treat. Cellular deformity, leading to structural changes, is clearly developed.

Unfortunately, prognosis for recovery at the sixth stage is slim. This is the point where medical intervention may briefly prolong life through drastic measures such as life support. In the sixth stage a *kapha* person may have cancer in the lymph system and in multiple organs and tissues. A *pitta* person may have paralysis from a severe stroke. A *vata* person may suffer from advanced Alzheimer's, not even recognizing his/her own family. It is at this stage that individuals or their families must make agonizing decisions about quality of life and what actions to take, medical or otherwise.

However, hope is always present. While statistically the advanced stage of disease almost always leads to death, there are exceptions. Even if the physical disease process cannot be reversed, many people at this stage experience deep emotional and spiritual healing by coming to terms with many of the issues in their lives.

The purpose of this book is to raise awareness around the first three stages of the disease process. These stages, before any disease can be diagnosed, are the stages during which you say: "My doctor says I'm fine, so why do I feel so bad?" These are the stages when many of the principles presented in this book can most easily be applied for self-healing. These same principles can certainly be used to treat advanced imbalances of the *doshas,* but that is beyond the scope of this book.

Knowledge of the pathogenic process is important, because it allows you to check the spread of disturbed *doshas* before a disease develops. "The key is awareness. The more you are alert to how your mind, body and emotions are reacting to changing circumstances, the more you are aware of your constitution and the moment-to-moment choices you can make to maintain health, the less opportunity you create for becoming sick."[4]

Conceptually, then, the keys to understanding your own conditions lie in becoming aware of the qualities in your life that are affecting your health, the qualities associated with "too much" or "too little" as manifested in the doshas. Either "too much" or "too little," excess or its opposite, leads to imbalances. Most illness is based on excess, and prolonged excess leads to accumulation, aggravation, overflow or spreading, infiltration, manifestation and destruction. The earlier intervention takes place by introducing opposite qualities, the more quickly balance is restored.

The strength of one's individual constitution, intimately connected with immunity, resistance to disease, is the most important factor in maintaining optimal health. The aim of this book is to help promote and restore this natural state of balance and sense of well-being of body, mind and consciousness.

What We Are Treating: Vata, Pitta and Kapha

Western medicine treats people who have diagnosable diseases. For example, it treats kidney diseases, such as kidney failure, nephritis, metabolic and congenital kidney disorders, urinary tract infections and obstructions, etc. It does not treat kidney energy imbalances. It does not treat *vata, pitta,* or *kapha.* Eastern medicine does not treat the diseases diagnosed in Western medicine. It treats imbalances in the *doshas* that underlie all diseases. All of the recommendations we make are aimed at helping you establish the proper balance of *vata, pitta* and *kapha* for you as an individual, regardless of where you are in the disease process. Remember you are in a state of balance when your current relationship of *vata-pitta-kapha* matches your basic constitution.

At no time in this book do we treat disease. Sometimes when we are dealing with clients clinically we use the language of symptoms and Western diagnosis to discuss their concerns. We do so because Ayurvedic terms are not widely understood. For example, there are five different types of *vata, pitta* and *kapha,* and these types interact with one another in complicated ways. It is meaningless for us to tell a client that excess *tarpaka kapha* is blocking *sadhaka pitta.* Instead, we would describe early symptoms of this blockage as a sense of heaviness in the head, difficulty in completing mental tasks, difficulty focusing attention due to lack of clarity in thinking, etc. At later stages we might describe depression or more advanced stages of diseases which cause tumors. One earlier stage does not inevitably lead to other more complicated stages. And there is not a one to one correlation between Ayurvedic and Western diagnosis. There is simply a failure of the English language to describe the more complicated forms of *vata, pitta* and *kapha.* Therefore, we must rely on the "language of the West," the "language" of symptoms and diseases.

Who Is in Control Here?
Does Food Control You or Do You Control Your Food Choices?

In the early chapters *vata, pitta* and *kapha* were described in terms of their qualities. *Vata* qualities are dry, light, mobile, cool, dispersing, clear, subtle and rough. *Pitta* qualities are hot, penetrating, light, mobile, oily, liquid and smelly (sour, pungent odor). *Kapha* qualities are wet, heavy, oily, sweet, dense, soft, static, cold, slow and slimy (like mucus).

You can perceive everything that happens to you both externally and internally in terms of qualities. The room you are in may be too hot, too cold, too dry, too humid or just right. Your food may be too oily, too dry, too wet, too hot, too cold, etc. Emotionally you may be feeling empty and dry, full and abundant, light or heavy. Your spirit may feel drained from burn-out, or nurtured and nourished after a time-out.

Food also has qualities. Fat, salt, sugar, red meat and most grains are heavy. Chilis and food high in acid content, such as tomatoes, oranges, grapefruit and lemons, are all hot. Salads and vegetables (without oil and sauces/dressings) are light. The qualities of the food you eat affect your *doshas* by increasing or decreasing the qualities associated with *vata, pitta* and *kapha.*

Rather than attempt to relate every single food on our extensive food lists to its qualities, we have chosen to simply list foods by category in an appendix, indicating whether they increase or decrease *vata, pitta* or *kapha.* If you use a common sense approach, with experience you can begin to discern which foods are related most closely to your particular imbalances. For example, if you have *kapha* problems pertaining to excessive weight, you must be careful in your use of oils and grains (your body will generate energy from the grains and readily convert any excess grain into fat, instead of using the excess fat you already have as energy). If, however, you are primarily concerned about liquid retention, which is also *kapha,* you need to pay attention to salt and foods that are high in liquid content, such as melons and summer squash.

There is often an inverse relationship between *vata* and *kapha* foods. Dry and light foods—such as raw salads and foods without any oil, water or other lubrication—naturally increase the dry quality of *vata*. Those that are wet, oily and heavy—such as sauces and dairy, meats and desserts—naturally increase *kapha*. The foods then that generally decrease *vata* increase *kapha*. Excess *vata* needs lubrication, excess *kapha* needs dryness. If you are a person who has imbalances in *vata* and *kapha*, select which one you want to work on first and focus on the other secondarily. In some cases both can be dealt with at the same time. For example, a person who is highly nervous (*vata*) and overweight (*kapha*) might lubricate with massage oils while reducing internal oil consumption. The external oil calms *vata* and the reduced internal oil helps calm *kapha* and promote weight loss.

Since the dietary lists in the appendix are general in nature and apply to the whole range of *vata, pitta* and *kapha* imbalances, you do need to apply some discrimination in determining which food modifications you wish to make. What works best is slow gradual change, unless you have a life-threatening illness that requires complete dedication to radical dietary change.

Food choices are not always based on rational, intellectual decisions. They are often based on emotions. Often foods are selected for the gratification and comfort they seem to give. Sometimes they are chosen simply out of habit or convenience. There are people who eat for comfort and others who refrain from eating, often because that gives them feelings of "control."

Telling a person who is not in balance to refrain from foods that have the same qualities as the imbalance invariably leads to the same response—"But what will I eat?" There are foods that tend to have the most negative impact on each *dosha*. Those who are high in *vata* like raw foods and foods that tend to create gas and "spaciness"—beans, broccoli, cauliflower, cabbage, brussel sprouts and any raw or juiced vegetables. They easily become "space cadets" who have a great deal of trouble sticking to any routine, especially one that involves diet. Their eating patterns are likely to be erratic and changeable like the mobile, dispersing and more subtle qualities of *vata*. They may even have a fear of oil, generally expressed as an obsession with becoming "too fat."

Pitta imbalances, in contrast, tend to be connected with hot, light, mobile and oily qualities. The *pitta* person will be drawn to foods that have these same qualities—peppers and chilis, hot spices, acidic foods such as citrus and vinegars, and fermented foods such as beer, wine and pickles. Try to remove these foods too quickly and those with *pitta* imbalances become irritable and angry.

Kapha imbalances reflect heaviness, oiliness, density and slowness. Those with *kapha* imbalances are drawn to foods that are heavy, oily, dense and slow to digest—wheat, dairy, meat, anything fried, most sauces and gravies, and almost all desserts. Remove these foods too quickly and those with *kapha* imbalances feel deprived and depressed.

The cardinal rule then is to make slow gradual change. We can speak from personal experience. When Shoshana went to an Ayurvedic practitioner for the first time in 1992, she was told she would need a *kapha* reducing diet and should give up dairy, wheat, heavy meats and desserts. "But what will I eat?" she said, quite typically. She looked in her refrigerator. There was milk, cheese, meat, bread, blue cheese salad dressing and a few vegetables for salads. Over a period of months she began with decreasing the amount of dairy and meat. She added more vegetables. In the spring of 1993 she started paying attention to the kind of oils she used and learned to make sauces that were not filled with oil and dairy. In 1994 she gave up her microwave, because it kills the life force in food. She also stopped buying processed food, including frozen dinners. By 1995 she followed a largely Ayurvedic diet, except for the presence of coffee, alcohol and some sweets in her diet. In 1995 she greatly decreased coffee from about seven to eight cups per day to one or two. In 1997 she began taking vitamin/mineral supplements regularly after courses in naturopathy convinced her they would be helpful. In 1998 she added essential fatty acids. Over the years she slowly decreased her intake of wheat until she discovered how she could enjoy and stay free of congestion. At present she eats almost any fruit but is careful about those with high sugar content, because she has a tendency to be hypoglycemic. She does drink wine and coffee occasionally and enjoys both as a special treat. She no longer eats sweet desserts or fast food. Her changes have come over a period of seven years. This is not to say that everyone needs to take seven years to make basic dietary changes. Rather it is to say that everyone goes at his/her own speed. In

Shoshana's case she made changes as her knowledge increased and as they fitted into her lifestyle.

Shoshana began making changes in her diet to relieve her congestion. As it began to disappear, she tuned in more carefully to her body's reactions to different foods and made further dietary changes. She has tried vegetarianism twice in her life, both times leading to medical diagnoses of severe malnutrition. At present the meat Shoshana eats is primarily poultry, because she is allergic to almost all seafood and has little taste for red meat. While most of her meals are freshly prepared at home, she enjoys dining out in restaurants that serve fresh food.

Awareness: What Do You Eat?
And What Gets in the Way of Change?

As you think about making dietary changes, your thoughts are likely to turn to food preferences. However, your success or failure in making changes will be determined in large part by lifestyle or even psychological factors. We suggest that your first task is to clearly and honestly look at how you lead your life and how food fits into your life. What do you generally do from morning until bedtime? Are your responsibilities so extensive that there is no time for you? Can you get even ten minutes of alone time? How much control do you have over what you eat? What do you in fact eat? There can be some surprising answers to these questions. As you pursue your personal journey of self-discovery, do not be embarrassed. Many people do not have conscious awareness of their food selections or even how they lead their lives. The fact that your choices have been less than perfect should be no surprise, given any imbalances you may be experiencing. What is important is that you become aware of what you do so that you can then have choice.

Let's look at some examples of patterns that can easily get in the way of change, and how the people in these examples altered their patterns to improve their health.

Dore suffered from severe fatigue. She almost did not return for a follow-up appointment, because she just could not follow the recommendations, especially the dietary ones. She did, however, reluctantly return. Together we examined the reasons she found follow-up difficult and discovered, much to our surprise, that it was because she literally did not eat regular meals—and all recommendations had been made around eating such meals. Prior to her follow-up session, Dore really was not aware that she wasn't eating regular meals. Dore's career was in sales, and she spent much time in her car. Rather than completely change her sporadic eating schedule, it was suggested that she purchase a cooler and keep it on the front seat of her car, which she did. Into it went nutritional drinks and food that provided her with balanced nutrients. Now she could graze and meet her dietary needs.

Was this an ideal approach? No, but Dore found this approach worked for her. With this relatively easy change in her eating habits, she did in fact deal successfully with her fatigue problem. Change occurs most easily when you start from "where you are" rather than from "where you think you ought to be." Dore was successful when she took that approach.

Brian ate almost all of his meals in fast food restaurants. In his job he traveled a regular route and knew all the fast food places along the way, ranging from burger places to Mexican and Chinese. We made a list of the kinds of restaurants he frequented and then planned the best foods for him to eat at each one. Brian was able to implement these changes.

Joan generally skipped breakfast, had yogurt for lunch and frozen dinners at night. In her case, we added a breakfast drink, light entrees for lunch and fruit snacks. For dinner we selected the kinds of frozen dinners and convenience foods that would be best for her needs.

Shawn was a teenager brought against his will by two exasperated parents. Shawn was so fatigued he was unable to function in school. He loved basketball but was too tired to play. His concentration was so poor he really could not study. His parents were on his back all the time. Since he was almost non-functional, his self-esteem was low. To say his life was a mess is an understatement. While clients are welcome to have others present in our sessions, I (Shoshana) asked the parents to remain in the waiting room while Shawn and I explored the nature of his problems. Shawn did not live on food. He lived on Pepsi and sugar. He drank three 64 ounce containers of Pepsi per day, at a minimum. His sugar intake in addition to the sugar in Pepsi was considerable. Shawn started by deciding how much change he was willing to try in order to gain energy. The first month he cut his Pepsi intake in half. The next month he halved it again. By the end of three months he was drinking one Pepsi per day. In the meantime, we added food to his diet, including a greens drink. Within three or four months, Shawn was doing his homework and playing basketball—and he was quite proud of himself for being able to make the decisions he made and stick with them. His parents still wish he'd eliminate all Pepsi and sugar from his diet, but Shawn is satisfied that he has found an approach that works for him.

In none of the above cases did the individuals make extreme changes and, because of that, they were successful in improving their health. *The most important thing is to start from where you are and do those things that are workable for you.* As you become successful, you can go for more. Often people are satisfied simply to have their symptoms disappear. However, others want to maximize their health, which involves going beyond getting rid of symptoms. As a first step, we suggest the following basic process.

Step 1: Become aware of what you are eating and doing—and be honest about it. Do you incorporate private downtime for yourself as well as exercise time? Look at what you do to lower stress and ask yourself if it works in the long run. If you are relying on alcohol or drugs for relaxation, you need to deal with the fact that they are depressants, provide only temporary relief, and create problems of their own. If you use food for comfort, be aware that usually leads to obesity. If you exercise compulsively, know that can cause your nervous system to go on overload. What you are now doing is related to the symptoms that are causing you discomfort, if not pain. Nothing happens in a vacuum. It may have taken a long time for you to get to your current state, and it may take a long time for you to return to a healthier state. Much depends on how much effort you are willing to make and how far along you are in the disease process.

Step 2: Begin by improving your diet in the easiest way possible for you, selecting a change that fits into your current lifestyle. Start with simple dietary changes. There is no dietary approach that works for all people. The first step is to get the right categories of food into your body—fruits, vegetables, grains, proteins. The next step is to get the right kinds of foods within each category to lower particular *doshas*.

Step 3: Pick the changes you are willing to make and make them gradually, selecting those with the highest probability of success. Pick a change on a planned schedule. For some, a change a week is not too much. For others, a change a month is pushing it. Move at your own pace, but know the more quickly and thoroughly you are able to make changes, the more quickly symptoms will disappear and balance will be restored.

Review the food list in the appendix. Use those foods that reduce your kind of imbalance as your shopping list. Start limiting the quantity and frequency of foods on the "no-no" list that you feel quite attached to. Don't try to work on all desired changes at the same time. Almost anything can be enjoyed occasionally in moderation.

Step 4: Congratulate yourself for any progress you make—and refrain from beating up on yourself when you are less than perfect. Most of us have negative thought patterns we fall into automatically. When we are down on ourselves, change comes only with difficulty. It's always helpful to acknowledge success.

Rose pretended that she was quite selective in her diet. She was selective. She chose everything with salt, sugar and oil, and she ate lots of each. When she became obese, she did not connect it to her eating. She believed that being kind to herself meant indulging herself. As a result, her health decreased and her weight increased. Rose's health will continue to deteriorate, until she is willing to give up her self-deceptions.

In contrast, David freely enjoys a taste of almost everything in life. He watches his diet carefully. If he eats something that is not on his approved food list, he asks himself if it is worth the price he know he must pay. As long as his occasions of indulgence are infrequent, his health stays in excellent condition.

Step 5: Refrain from excuse making. So many times we put ourselves at the bottom of our priority list, postponing our personal needs and desires until we have finished something, or achieved some goal, or we do not take time to care for ourselves. We act as if we are machines that need only an occasional oil and grease job, with no other maintenance. Such an approach to ourselves can work in the short run but it *never* works in the long run. Consider where you are on your priority list and, if necessary, make some changes. *If you do not change your priorities, then you will experience the negative consequences of inaction.*

Jean was married to her job, placing it above care for herself, until she became acutely aware of some negative consequences. While she loved to exercise, she worked at least 12 hours a day, usually six days a week and part-time on the seventh day. By the time she did her shopping, housecleaning and errands, there was little time to exercise. She joined a gym and enjoyed going there, but seldom got to it. Then she started experiencing various aches and pains. Her upper body strength, never strong to begin with, became quite weak. She began to lose flexibility. One day she simply acknowledged to herself that the day of reckoning was upon her. She would either have to "use it or lose it." She asked herself how she could change her work schedule so that exercise could be included, and then she made the change. She did the same thing with her eating. While she had watched her diet carefully, she had tended to eat in restaurants once or twice a day, which meant no control over the kinds of fats used in food preparation. With planning she was able to come up with easy to prepare menus for home cooking, as well as with low fat restaurant food she could have when she ate out.

It is not lack of intellectual understanding of what we should do in behalf of better health that stands in our way most of the time. Do you know anyone, for example, who seriously believes unlimited sugar consumption is good for him/her? No, it is emotional attachments, old habits, and deepseated self-defeating belief systems that stand in our way.

Step 6: Check your imbalance indicators regularly by re-examining the markings on your face, tongue, eyes, ears, hands and feet (and pulse if you can) periodically. When you take steps to change, your body actually does respond, and progress can be seen by observing the indicators. Lines change. In particular, check your tongue. Markings on it can change rapidly. Facial and other markings change more slowly.

Joyce had deep anxiety marks on her forehead, but began adding lubricating oils to her otherwise *vata* aggravating diet of raw vegetables and beans. In addition, she took calming herbs and learned relaxation techniques and yoga. Her forehead lines are now quite faint. Carl had deep vertical lines between his brows, indicating imbalances in his liver and spleen. He changed his diet to cooler foods, stopped exercising at the hottest time of day, stayed away from hot tubs and saunas, and learned relaxation techniques. He no longer has those lines.

Change is possible and can involve many lifestyle changes, including diet. Now let us look at actual dietary choices, starting with where to begin.

Getting on the Right Track

It is not clear to most people what makes up a basic healthy diet. And even those who know find it difficult to obtain needed nutrients, because of the prevalence of fast food, frozen and other processed foods, as well as restaurant foods that rely heavily on fat, salt and sugar for flavoring and preservatives for shelf life. Recognizing that this is the case, we make the following observations. First, it is important to know what constitutes a good basic food plan. Next, it is important to acquire awareness about the effect of convenience foods that are laden with sugar, refined carbohydrates (bread, pasta, muffins, etc.), fats and salt. Convenience foods produce a host of symptoms you have probably experienced but have not connected to the way you are eating. Once you alter eating habits to include more nutrients from the basic food groups, you can refine your food selections to decrease foods that create problems with your *doshas*. Finally, it is important for you to gain awareness of the relationship between your food selection patterns, your *doshic* imbalances and your blood type.

Whatever your starting point, progress needs to be made toward a more wholesome way of eating that includes the right food categories: fruits, vegetables, grains and proteins. Given individual variance, most people will do quite well if they eat the following foods daily:

Basic Dietary Needs

Fruits	2-3 servings per day of fruit or juice (1/2 cup = 1 serving)
Vegetables	2-5 servings per day (1/2 cup = 1 serving)
Grains	3-5 servings per day (1/2 cup rice or other grain = 1 serving; 1 cup pasta = 1 serving; 1 slice bread or 1/2 bagel = 1 serving)
Protein	2-3 servings (not more than 4-6 oz. each) of chicken, fish, meat, tofu, tempeh or other protein source

In addition to the above, your body needs plenty of antioxidants to cleanse toxins or free radicals from your system. These are found in Vitamins A, C and E as well as in all the bitter tasting greens such as alfalfa, wheatgrass and blue-green algae. Because bitter greens are too bitter for most people, we recommend taking them as a green drink or together in a few capsules. Shoshana's favorite recipe is:

Greens Drink

1 heaping teaspoon of green powder
1 cup juice (dilute if you tend to get hypoglycemic reactions)
1 tsp. flaxseed oil
1 tsp. lecithin
Place in blender to create a refreshing smoothie.

In addition, we recommend a good multi-vitamin/mineral supplement (select one that is high in B-Complex if you are under stress), Vitamin C, and a Calcium/Magnesium supplement daily. In addition, we recommend a supplementation of essential fatty acids, in particular Omega-3s. Possible sources for these are listed in the appendix.

Pointing out what you ought to do in an ideal way is the easy part. The more difficult part is beginning to make the changes. In a separate appendix we have prepared ways for you to modify your diet regardless of your dietary lifestyle. We start from the idea that any change in a positive direction is better than no change. While there are specific foods for managing the *doshas*, you must first be sure you are getting the essential nutrients into your body. Only then can you turn to improving your diet and lifestyle to overcome doshic imbalances. We make suggestions about several dietary lifestyles: diets that rely largely on fast food, frozen food, restaurants, quick meals (cans, packages, and other pre-prepared foods) and fresh food. A busy person who grabs a quick burger and fries at noon is not likely to stop doing that in order to take a bag lunch of salad, cut veggies, and a sandwich on homemade bread. Improvements can be incorporated in any of these lifestyles and, the more you invest in your health, the more you will move over time toward fresh foods.

Finally, a word about the non-nutrients—coffee, other caffeine, alcohol, chips, desserts. If you eat a healthy diet, particularly one accompanied by the suggested supplements, cravings for the non-nutrients will begin to lessen. In the meantime, start moving toward a path of moderation. To help mitigate against the negative effects of caffeinated drinks such as coffee and tea, add a pinch of cardamom, ginger, nutmeg and cinnamon to your drinks. For those of you who like lattes and/or flavored drinks, try this recipe:

Flavor Recipe for Coffee or Tea

Prepare in advance this mixture to be added to hot drinks.

1/3 cup ground cardamom	1/3 cup ground ginger
1/8 cup ground nutmeg	1/8 cup ground cinnamon

Add the above mixture up to 1/2 teaspoon per cup, depending on your taste, to a cup of coffee or tea.

As with coffee and tea, alcohol can be enjoyed in moderation, unless you have a tendency toward addiction. The type of alcohol that is best for each *dosha* is included in the food list in the appendix.

Common Dietary Problems: The Ups and Downs of Energy and Other Challenges

There is much advice available on what kinds of foods are best for you. There seems to be a diet for every imaginable condition, and very little guidance to help you determine what is best for you. Our experience with many people has convinced us that the Ayurvedic approach to eating is viable and healthy. But before you can use this approach successfully, you need to know about patterns that get in the way of healthy eating.

Some of the most common complaints we hear are:[1]

Fatigue	Depression	Low pain tolerance
Restlessness	Impulsiveness	Tearfulness
Confusion	Short attention	Low self-esteem
Memory loss	Feeling scattered	Overly sensitive
Concentration loss	Emotionalism	Isolation
High frustration	Suicidal tendencies	Hopelessness
Irritability	Sweet cravings	Sugar cravings
Easily angered	Craving bread, pasta, cereals	Easily overwhelmed

It is easy to slip into a dietary pattern that relies on sugar, refined carbohydrates (bread, pasta, cereal, muffins, etc.), fat, caffeine, and even alcohol for energy. Such a pattern creates the above problems, due to imbalances in blood sugar, serotonin and beta-endorphins, particularly for those who are sugar sensitive. Sugar sensitive people crave the above foods, but eating them can lead to huge swings in their blood sugar, so much so that they alternate between wild energy surges and crashing. They reach for one of the above foods for more energy followed by another surge and another crash. The pattern becomes endless, eventually leading to fatigue, depression and many of the other complaints listed above.

If this pattern is present in your life, you may find it helpful to read Kathleen DesMaisons' *Potatoes Not Prozac*. She presents clear, useful information about what is taking place. Most important, she provides a highly workable step by step plan that can change your life through proper eating, and she does this is a manner that leaves you completely in control.[2]

The need to break the refined carbohydrate, sugar, oil, caffeine, alcohol cycle (or any part of these that applies to you) is the first step.

Once you have accomplished that, you can begin to focus on your *doshic* imbalances. Take it in steps: first the breaking of the cycle, then the modifications that help rebalance your *doshas*.

Eating to Rebalance Vata, Pitta or Kapha

As you examine the imbalances that are causing you problems, keep in mind that you do not have to give up everything you love to eat, but you do need to make changes. *For those foods that increase a dosha that is too high but which you feel you cannot live without, cut down on the quantity you eat and the frequency of eating them.*

• *Vata imbalances*: Cut back on foods that create gas, and add lubrication to your diet. If you eat salad, use salad dressing that contains a good oil, such as olive oil. Avoid saturated fat from meats and hydrogenated oils of all kinds (including those in margarine). If you feel you must have a gas producing food such as broccoli, cook it and add a little clarified butter (ghee) or oil to help eliminate the gas. To beans, add herbs such as hing or Asafetida (an Ayurvedic powder that tastes a little like garlic) or epazote (a plant used commonly in the Southwest for gas) or even Bean-o. Try soaking beans overnight and changing the water before cooking. Stay away from dry, raw foods.

• *Pitta imbalances*: Cut back on hot, acidic and fermented foods. Be wary of Mexican foods, Chinese Szechwan, hot spices, orange juice and other citrus fruits, vinegars and pickles, all widely available foods that increase *pitta*. Become acquainted with the spices on the dietary list for *pitta* that can take the place of hot spices and use them freely. In cooking meals at home, this is easy. In eating out, don't hesitate to find an herbal mixture that can be carried with you in a shaker and add it to anything that tastes too bland.

• *Kapha imbalances*: Salty chips, desserts, dairy (especially cheese and ice cream) and fried, oily foods are the worst culprits. You can begin by substituting low fat cheese and dairy products, and low salt baked chips (such as baked tortilla chips). You can also cut back on high calorie desserts, finding low calorie substitutes. However, this is just a beginning. Next, start adding hot spices to your food, such as cayenne, pepper and chiles, to improve your digestion. Add slowly and in moderate amounts that do not jolt you or burn your taste buds. If you have water retention, watch out for foods with high water content, such as melons and squashes. If you have congestion, avoid dairy and wheat products until you clear up.

High *vata* is reduced more quickly when dietary changes are combined with an established daily routine. A daily routine grounds *vata,* and leads to a more regular, consistent effort. In addition to diet, high *pitta* responds to anything that cools—being in a cool room, taking a cool bath, eating cooling food, doing things that cool emotional heat, such as relaxation exercises, meditation and yoga. *Kapha* imbalances respond best to vigorous exercise combined with diet. For imbalances in any of the three *doshas*, diet alone is unlikely to be enough.

What do you do when all of your doshas are in a state of imbalance? The answer is simple. Begin anywhere but don't try to do all things at once. *Vata* is changeable by its very nature. Its qualities are those of movement and mobility. Therefore, on the physical level *vata* imbalances are usually the easiest to change, especially in the early phases of the disease process. However, because those with high *vata* tend to dislike routine, resistance to change can set in easily. *Kapha* by nature is slow, dense and heavy. Therefore, *kapha* imbalances usually take the longest to correct. Study your symptoms, correlate them with the indicators, and select the course that is easiest for you.

Move from the obvious to the subtle. In the beginning, it is enough that you just eat the right nutrients—grains, proteins, fruits and vegetables. Any fruits are better than no fruits. Any vegetables are better than no vegetables. Any grains are better than no grains. Any protein you like is better than no protein. Cutting down on salt is better that high salt, even if you do not switch to better kinds of salt. Cutting back on sugar is better than high sugar, but eating the right sweetener for your constitution is better still. The exception to this is with oils. Most oils used in cooking are harmful to your body, because they lead to the storage of waste in your cells. This is discussed in more detail in Chapter Ten. Only by eating the right oils, including omega-3s, do you promote elimination of waste. Once you are eating the right nutrients, begin selecting more of the right foods for your constitution and imbalances.

Eating Right for Your Constitution:
The Doshas and Blood Type

The relationship between common problems and a diet consisting primarily of sugar, refined carbohydrates, caffeine, oil, etc. clearly leads to symptoms associated with *doshic* imbalance. These problems are readily corrected through dietary changes, particularly when foods that correct imbalances for *vata, pitta* and *kapha* become a regular part of your diet. However, while these problems readily occur in the initial stages of the disease process, not all problems are related to these factors.

The correlation between blood type and diet has become a topic of interest in recent years, because of the work of Peter D'Adamo, the author of *Eat Right 4 Your Type*. Nutrients are carried to our individual cells by our blood. Clearly there is a chemical relationship between our blood and the nutrients. According to D'Adamo, the type of relationship is determined in part by the type of blood we have. There are four basic blood types: A, B, AB and O. A and B are incompatible. If you give type A a blood transfusion of type B blood or vice versa, a severe reaction will result that can sometimes lead to death. Many foods are similar in structure to blood types. If a type A person eats food that is similar in structure to type B blood, the type A blood will produce antibodies that will attach to the food, or to any incompatible foreign substances (antigens) that invade the body. The purpose of the antibodies is to neutralize the effects of incompatible antigens or substances. This process is called agglutination. Agglutination causes cells, viruses, parasites and bacteria to stick together for easier removal from the body. This system can be quite helpful in warding off disease.[3] If however you eat foods that are incompatible with your blood, agglutination occurs more slowly, because incompatible proteins, called lectins, start the clumping process, target an organ or bodily system, and begin to slowly agglutinate blood cells in that area.[4]

Because of agglutination, it becomes important to know which foods most readily affect blood type. According to Ayurveda, this determination can be made by knowing your basic constitution, even if you are not aware of your blood type, because Ayurveda relates *doshas* to blood type.

Blood Type and Dosha[5]	
Blood Type	**Dominant Doshas**
A	Vata, Pitta
B	Kapha, Pitta
AB	Vata, Kapha
O	Pitta

Peter D'Adamo presents food lists identifying the foods to be avoided by each blood type. In comparing D'Adamo's lists with Dr. Lad's *vata, pitta, kapha* lists, we found a high correlation.[6] A person whose basic constitution is *pitta* and blood type is A will do well avoiding those foods which increase *pitta*. A *vata* with blood type A will do well avoiding those foods which increase *vata*. Those who already follow the D'Adamo plan can readily incorporate an Ayurvedic approach. The primary difference is that Ayurveda focuses on the qualities that are out of balance, and links the **qualities** to *vata, pitta* and *kapha*. To reestablish balance of any *dosha* requires the presence of its opposite quality and is an ongoing process of change. If your constitution is *vata* but you are too high in *kapha*, steps must be taken to bring balance back to *kapha* regardless of blood type. However, if you are taking blood type into consideration, you simply select those foods from your blood type list that do not aggravate *kapha*. Because of the many possible variations of *vata, pitta* and *kapha*, the above table relates to dominant *doshas* only. They do not hold true 100 percent of the time.

The possible inter-relationship of these two approaches to constitution is worthy of further research. It may be possible, for example, to predict where disease is most likely to occur in an individual by knowing the relationships of blood type, the difference in basic constitution, current imbalances and dietary intake.

Ayurvedic dietary guidelines are extensive. They are located at the back of the book in a separate appendix. Study them and select the foods that are known to reduce the qualities you are attempting to bring back into balance. Use the lists for your food shopping.

Exercise

The right food choices are of paramount importance for good health. However, without proper exercise, the picture is incomplete. Although initially any form of exercise is better than no exercise, there are general guidelines for each dosha. People with high *vata* are naturally attracted to exercises that provoke *vata* by jarring the joints: running, skiing, bicycling, some aerobics. However, over time those with *vata* imbalances do best when they select exercise that does not pound their joints because they easily suffer from joint related problems. For them weights, yoga, t'ai chi, swimming and exercise machines are better.

People with high *pitta* are naturally attracted to exercises that make them sweat: tennis, basketball, hockey, exercising at the hottest time of day, etc. They also do better with things such as yoga, t'ai chi, swimming, weight and exercise machines and walking.

Those with high *kapha* prefer to sit as spectators or to do something simple such as swimming or water aerobics. They need to sweat and move. Walking is excellent for any constitution. See page 229 for more information about exercise.

Yoga. If you have seen pictures or videos or watched people do yoga but have never experienced it yourself, you are in for a surprise. It often looks as if the person is doing nothing other than placing the body in a certain position. When you try to do a pose yourself, you will discover that it is an intensive, rigorous form of exercise, but gentle enough for those who may have health restrictions. How well you can move your body into the optimal position is called "going into the pose." The rule is that you pay attention and move your body to the edge of resistance. If you are huffing, puffing, groaning or in pain, you have gone too far. Back off. The goal is not to force yourself into the optimal position when your body is resisting. The goal is to work at the edge of resistance so that you learn to relax what is tight. Then you can move more deeply into a pose.

We highly recommend that you attend yoga classes conducted by someone with whom you are comfortable. If this is not possible, then arrange a few private lessons to learn the correct way to move your body into a pose. Otherwise you can hurt yourself. We recommend certain poses for *vata, pitta* or *kapha* imbalances. They are:

Yoga poses that decrease vata:

Plough, cobra, locust, yoga mudra, half wheel, knee-to-chest, head stand, corpse, mountain.

Yoga poses that decrease pitta:

Shoulder stand, half boat, bow, fish, half wheel, ear-to-knee, sheetali (inhaling through coiled tongue in open mouth), cobra, moon salutation.

Yoga poses that decrease kapha:

Palm tree, forward bend, half-spinal twist, boat, wheel, locust, lion, sun salutation.

Any good yoga teacher can show you how to do these poses in a way that doesn't hurt your body. Don't be discouraged with doing modifications. Unless you are extremely flexible, your body will not pretzel into any ideal form apart from application over a period of time. Breathing deeply in the poses relaxes the muscles and makes them easier.

Yoga simultaneously relaxes and invigorates, especially after an exhausting day at work. It also works on more subtle levels, often producing seemingly miraculous physical, mental and spiritual benefits. Points of resistance correlate with energy and physical blockages. Holding a pose while focusing on release not only relaxes muscles but also releases emotional, intellectual and spiritual blockages you may not have been aware of.

Tina had a severe case of cervical dysplasia that did not respond to any prescribed medications. She was quite concerned because dysplasia can become cancerous. Just days after an examination that confirmed the medications had been ineffective, Tina left for a vacation to a yoga retreat center where she did yoga several hours a day. One day she did a pose in which she laid her body a round ball so that her back and pelvis stretched open.

Much to her astonishment she felt a rush of energy pour out between her legs, and was so alarmed she left the class to be sure she had not urinated. The sense of flow was quite strong. When she went to her next workshop and sat in a chair, she felt the flow cease. The sense of

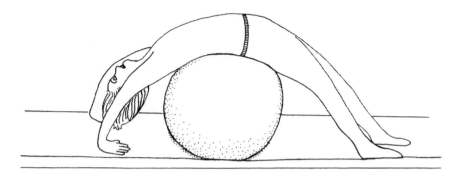

blockage was followed by extreme discomfort, even pain at times. After class she discussed her concern with the instructor, and for the next few days a mat was placed in each of her workshops for her to lie on. Prior to her next workshop, she was instructed to do the ball pose again while watching the flow of her thoughts, and then to write a paper on her experience. In the course of redoing the pose, she became aware of an emotional link between early childhood experiences and the onset of the blockage. The flow resumed and continued for several days. Tina experienced an enormous sense of relief. Several days after her return home, Tina went in for yet another lab test. There was no longer any indication of cervical dysplasia. She has now been free of abnormal cervical cells for 15 years. At the time of her release, Tina had never heard that yoga postures can produce healing in the body, but her personal experience was profound.

Most of us may not experience noticeable healing while doing yoga. If you never experience a healing effect, do not worry about it. Enjoy the relaxation and invigoration! If you choose to do yoga, start off gently about once a week and then add days gradually, until you are doing about 15 to 20 minutes of poses daily. Remember to begin with an instructor who can show you how to modify poses to "fit" your body so that you do not injure yourself.

CHAPTER 8

WHAT TO DO ABOUT WHAT GOES WRONG: TREATMENT

IN THIS CHAPTER we deal with the systems that are the sources of most people's health problems—the digestive, respiratory, circulatory, skeletal, skin, reproductive, and nervous systems. Each system outlines the *vata, pitta* and *kapha* symptoms most readily associated with *doshic* imbalances. We will outline the symptoms and suggest diet, herbs, exercise and yoga poses, which will help to bring balance to the respective *doshas.* The Ayurvedic herbs recommended come in tablets, capsules, ot tinctures that are safe and easy to self-administer. See the Resources Appendix for a source of Ayurvedic products.

This section is not meant to present comprehensive information on the use of western herbs for specific problems. There is an abundance of information available from other sources, such as Michael Tierra's *Planetary Herbology* and David Frawley's and Vasant Lad's *Yoga of Herbs,* both of which present western and eastern herbs with emphasis on their impact on the *doshas.* Our emphasis, of course, is on the use of traditional Ayurvedic approaches, especially food, Ayurvedic herbs, lifestyle and exercise. In general, *vata* and *pitta* imbalances respond to relaxants because they are calming, while *kapha* imbalances respond to stimulants to overcome the sluggish qualities of *kapha.*

There are many excellent Western oriented sources as well. We include some western herbs that are known to be useful for a wide variety of problems. Terry Willard's *Herbs: Their Clinical Uses,* S. Linenger, et al., *The Natural Pharmacy,* Michael Murray's *Encyclopedia of Nutritional Supplements,* Amanda McQuade Crawford's *Herbal Remedies for Women,* Joseph Pizzorno and Michael Murray's *Encyclopedia of Natural Medicine* all present a wide variety of herbs for common health problems.

With exercise there are general guidelines for each *dosha*. People with excessive *vata* need forms of exercise that are not jarring, especially to the skeletal system. That means replacing exercise such as jumping and running with forms that are centering and more gentle on the bones. People with excessive *pitta* need to exercise without becoming overheated, so it is best for them to exercise at cooler times of the day. People with excessive *kapha* need vigorous exercise that gets them moving and sweating. Within these contexts there are many varieties from which to choose.

In addition to suggestions for treatment presented in this chapter, a number of labs are now offering functional assessment tests. If you have a problem that does not respond to the protocols suggested in this book, you might consider finding a healthcare practitioner who can order appropriate tests for you. Lab information is included in the Resources appendix. Please be aware that these labs only deal with healthcare practitioners, and this information is included for you to give to your practitioner.

Digestive System		
Vata Symptoms	**Pitta Symptoms**	**Kapha Symptoms**
Gas	Inflammation	Malabsorption
Constipation	Heartburn	Water retention
Bloating	Indigestion	Obesity
Burping	Irritability	Sluggish digestion
Coldness	Mouth ulcers	Yeast
Nervousness	Sensitive teeth	Lack of appetite
Hard, small stools	Hot stools	Oily, heavy stools
Weight loss	Warm urine	Blockages: stones
Dehydration	Infections	Blockages: tumors
Dry hemorrhoids	Craves hot, acidic	Craves oil, sweet, salt
Colic		

Treatment for Vata Digestive Problems
Food Plan: Vata reducing. See the appendix.
Exercise: Vata yoga poses, walking, exercise machines, weights, swimming

Herbs: For all *doshas:* Cumin-coriander-fennel tea, Triphala, Ginger. *Vata* reducing herbs are generally calming, lubricating and tonifying. They include Chamomile, Peppermint and Lemon Balm. For gas, constipation and bloating, increase oil in the diet, especially clarified butter (also called *ghee*). Ginger tea from ginger root or powder with lemon and honey and ginger candy are also excellent.
Ayurvedic Formulas: Triphala, Hingvastak

Treatment for Pitta Digestive Problems
Food Plan: *Pitta* reducing. See the appendix.
Exercise: *Pitta* yoga poses, walking, exercise machines, weights, swimming
Herbs: For all *doshas:* Cumin-coriander-fennel tea, Triphala, Ginger. *Pitta* reducing herbs are calming, cooling and anti-inflammatory. They include Chamomile, Peppermint and Thyme. For indigestion, heartburn, acidity and diarrhea, use aloe vera gel, licorice, ginger tea made with fresh ginger root (powder is too heating) and cooked apples. Avoid foods that are hot and spicy such as chili and peppers, acidic such as orange juice and vinegars, or fermented such as beer and wine.
Ayurvedic Formulas: Digest Ease, Triphala

Treatment for Kapha Digestive Problems
Food Plan: *Kapha* reducing. See the appendix.
Exercise: *Kapha* yoga poses, walking, exercise machines, weights, aerobics, skiing
Herbs: For all *doshas:* Cumin-coriander-fennel tea, Triphala, Ginger. *Kapha* reducing herbs are stimulating, warming and increase digestion. They include Ginger tea made with powdered ginger, garlic, horseradish, mustard and mustard seeds. Cut back on oil (especially fried foods), sweets such as desserts and candy, and salty snacks such as chips.
Ayurvedic Formulas Trikatu, Trim Support (for weight problems) and Triphala.

Respiratory System		
Vata Symptoms	**Pitta Symptoms**	**Kapha Symptoms**
Clear mucus	Green/yellow mucus	Thick, white mucus
Dry cough	Warm chest	Wet cough
Shortness of breath		Sinus headache

Treatment for Vata Respiratory Problems

Food Plan: Vata reducing. See the Appendix.

Exercise: Vata yoga poses, walking, weights, exercise machines, swimming.

Herbs: For all *doshas,* licorice tea (unless there is high blood pressure), zinc lozenges, ginger tea with honey and lemon (lime for *pitta),* eucalyptus steam, Echinacea and Ayurvedic nose drops. For relaxation, lavender and chamomile tea or aromatherapy. With any congestion eliminate all dairy products except boiled milk, which does not produce mucus, and all wheat. Both dairy and wheat are mucous forming.

Vata Reducing Herbs: For dry cough use bananas with honey and lemon and any of the above listed herbs.

Ayurvedia Formula: Ayurvedic nose drops.

Treatment for Pitta Respiratory Problems

Food Plan: *Pitta* reducing. See the Appendix.

Exercise: *Pitta* yoga poses, walking, weights, exercise machines, swimming.

Pitta Reducing Herbs: For sore throat use boiled milk mixed with one-half teaspoon of turmeric. Also ginger tea with lime and honey, Vitamin C and Echinacea at the first sign of a cold. For those who are not vegetarians, try homemade chicken soup. Any of the above general herbs are helpful.

Ayurvedic Formula: Lung Formula, Ayurvedic nose drops.

Treatment for Kapha Respiratory Problems

Food Plan: Kapha reducing. See the Appendix.

Exercise: Kapha yoga poses, walking, weights, exercise machines, aerobics, skiing, bicycling.

Kapha Reducing Herbs: Same herbs as *pitta*.
Ayurvedic Formula: Lung Formula, Ayurvedic nose drops.

Circulatory/Heart Systems		
Vata Symptoms	**Pitta Symptoms**	**Kapha Symptoms**
Cold hands	Excessive body heat	Stagnation
Cold feet	High blood pressure	Broken blood vessels
Excessively low cholesterol	Excessive thirst	High cholesterol
Excessively low triglycerides	Bleeding nose	High triglycerides
Dry eyes	Bloodshot eyes	Moist, draining eyes
	Palpitations	Edema
		Enlarged lymph nodes
		Varicose veins

Treatment for Vata Circulatory/Heart Problems
Food Plan: Vata reducing diet.
Exercise: Yoga poses for vata, walking, weights, exercise machines, swimming.
Herbs: General herbs for all *doshas* include Hawthorn, Garlic, Ginkgo, Ginger, Rosemary, Dandelion, Flaxseeds or oil, essential fatty acids and Lavender. For *vata* use any of the above, plus Valerian.
Ayurvedic Formulas: Tranquil Mind, Yogaraj Guggulu.

Treatment for Pitta Circulatory/Heart Problems
Diet: Pitta reducing.
Exercise: Yoga poses for *pitta*, walking, weights, exercise machines, swimming.
Herbs: Pitta reducing herbs: Any of the above, especially Flaxseeds, essential fatty acids and Hawthorn.
Ayurvedic Formulas: Heart Formula, Liver Formula, Kaishore Guggulu

Treatment for Kapha Circulatory/Heart Problems
Food Plan: *Kapha* reducing.
Exercise: Yoga poses for *kapha*, walking, weights, exercise machines, aerobics, skiing, bicycling.
Herbs: Any of the above, especially Flaxseeds and essential fatty acids. Ginger, Marjoram and Cayenne compresses applied externally are also helpful.
Ayurvedic Formulas: Heart Formula, Triphala Guggulu

NOTE: For all persistent problems, especially those that are acute in nature and involve infections and inflammations, seek allopathic medical treatment if the symptoms become worse or persist.

Skeletal System		
Vata symptoms	**Pitta symptoms**	**Kapha symptoms**
Cracking joints	Bleeding gums	Swollen joints
Pain in joints/bones	Tooth decay	Unctuous joints
Receding gums		Extra teeth
Bone popping		Tissue calcification
Dryness in hair	Hair falling out	Oily hair
Split nails		
Slow healing of fractures and breaks		

Treatment for Vata Skeletal Problems
Food Plan: *Vata* reducing diet
Exercise: *Vata* yoga poses, walking, weights, exercise machines, swimming.
Herbs: Generally good for all *doshas* are Willow Bark, Castor Oil, Camphor (externally only). *Vata* reducing herbs include any of the above plus extra oil and supplemental calcium citrate and magnesium.
Ayurvedic Formulas: Yogaraj Guggulu, Bone Formula, Shilajit.

Treatment for Pitta Skeletal Problems
Food Plan: Pitta reducing.
Exercise: Pitta yoga poses, walking, weights, exercise machines, swimming.
Herbs: Pitta reducing herbs focus on reducing heat and inflammation. These include Devil's Claw, Yucca, Ginger, Black Cohosh, Mulberry and Turmeric. Calcium citrate and magnesium supplements are helpful.
Ayurvedic Formula: Kaishore Guggulu, Bone Formula, Liver Cleanser.

Treatment for Kapha Skeletal Problems
Diet: Kapha reducing.
Exercise: Kapha yoga poses, walking, weights, exercise machines, aerobics, skiing, bicycling.
Herbs: Kapha reducing herbs include any of the above general herbs, Garlic in food or caps and castor oil for fibroids and cysts.
Ayurvedic Formulas: Triphala Guggulu, Bone Formula.

Skin		
Vata symptoms	*Pitta symptoms*	*Kapha symptoms*
Dry skin	Hot skin	Oily skin
Dry mouth	Acne/pimples	Mouth watering
Sensitivity to noise	Red flushed skin	Fungus on skin
Cracked skin	Eczema/rashes	Thick skin
Dandruff	Bruises	Cysts
Fine goose pimples/ bumps	Body odor	
Flaking skin	Skin inflammations	
	Boils/abscesses	

Treatment for Vata Skin Problems
Food Plan: Vata reducing diet
Exercise: Vata yoga poses, walking, weights, exercise machines, swimming.

Herbs: Generally, relaxants such as Lavender, Chamomile, Lemon Balm are all helpful to the skin. In addition, Evening Primrose Oil is recommended. Vitamin B complex is helpful, also, particularly when the skin problem correlates with increased nervous tension or stress. *Vata* reducing herbs include lavender, chamomile and lemon balm as relaxants. For internal oleation use clarified butter (*ghee*) and essential fatty acids. Externally, massage with pure sesame oil (regular, not Chinese). Sesame oil is warming. Olive oil can be used during hot seasons, because it is cooling and is good for all three *doshas*. Use only raw unprocessed oils if possible.
Ayurvedic Formula: Triphala

Treatment for Pitta Skin Problems
Food Plan: Pitta reducing.
Exercise: Pitta yoga poses, walking, weights, exercise machines, swimming.
Herbs: Pitta reducing herbs include any of the above general herbs, particularly Lavender. Also Slippery Elm, Aloe Vera, Red Clover tea and Evening Primrose Oil are good. For compresses, consider Witchazel (1 tablespoon with 1 cup water) plus several drops of Lemon Balm and Lavender oil. Externally Tea Tree oil and Lavender, several drops each mixed with olive oil, is soothing to the skin. Tea Tree oil and several drops of Chamomile or Lavender oil prepared as a compress has an antiseptic, anti-inflammatory effect. Omega 3 and Omega 6 are also helpful.
Ayurvedic Formula: Liver Cleanser.

Treatment for Kapha Skin Problems
Food Plan: Kapha reducing.
Exercise: Kapha yoga poses, walking, weights, exercise machines, aerobics, skiing, bicycling.
Herbs: Kapha reducing herbs include any of the above general herbs, plus Garlic in food or caps and Castor Oil for fibroids and cysts. Calcium citrate and magnesium are helpful.
Ayurvedic Formula: Triphala, Triphala Guggulu

Reproductive System: Female		
Vata Symptoms	**Pitta symptoms**	**Kapha symptoms**
Dry vagina	Hot flashes	Excessive secretions
Scanty, short periods	Heavy hot flow	Heavy flow, clotting
Cramps which move around	Sharp, intense cramps	Dull cramps
		Fibrocystic breast changes

Reproductive System: Male		
Vata Symptoms	**Pitta symptoms**	**Kapha symptoms**
Lack of sperm	Testicular inflammation	Excessive virility
Impotence	Prostate inflammation	Enlarged prostate
Premature ejaculation		
Low libido		

Treatment for Vata Reproductive Problems
Food Plan: Vata reducing diet.
Exercise: Vata yoga poses, walking, weights, exercise machines, swimming.
Herbs: General for all *doshas,* use Evening Primrose oil, boiled milk with Turmeric, and relaxants such as Chamomile and Lemon Balm teas or essential oils. For women Geranium and Rose oil mixed with massage oil can be used for massage or added to bath water. Yarrow or Nettle tea can be helpful. *Vata* reducing herbs for women include Cramp Bark, Valerian and any of the above general oils. Saw Palmetto is particularly helpful for male prostate problems. Omega 3 and Omega 6 are also helpful.
Ayurvedic formula: Women's Support / Men's Support

Treatment for Pitta Reproductive Problems
Food Plan: Pitta reducing diet.
Exercise: Pitta yoga poses, walking, weights, exercise machines, swimming.

Herbs: In addition to the general herbs, *pitta* reducing herbs for women include Chaste Tree Berry.

Ayurvedic Formula: Women's Support / Men's Support

Treatment for Kapha Reproductive Problems

Food Plan: Kapha reducing diet.

Exercise: Kapha yoga poses, walking, weights, exercise machines, aerobic, skiing, bicycling.

Herbs: Kapha reducing herbs for women include Cramp Bark and any of the above general herbs.

Ayurvedic formula: Women's Support / Men's Support

For men: Saw Palmetto is useful for prostate problems as is Horsetail for all *doshas.* In addition, Ashwaghanda and Men's Support are recommended for low libido and sexual dysfunction.

Urinary System		
Vata Symptoms	**Pitta Symptoms**	**Kapha Symptoms**
Incontinence	Urinary tract infections	Excessive urine
Scanty urine	Dark urine	Obstruction
	Inflammation	Urine retention
	Acidosis	Cloudy urine

Treatment for Vata Urinary Problems

Food Plan: Vata reducing diet.

Exercise: Swimming, exercise machines, walking, *vata* yoga poses, weights.

Herbs: Increase water intake.

Ayurvedic Formulas: Kidney Formula, Yogaraj Guggulu.

Treatment for Pitta Urinary Problems

Food Plan: Pitta reducing diet.

Exercise: Swimming, exercise machines, walking, yoga, weights.

Herbs: Cranberry, Uva Ursi, Echinacea, Goldenseal, Sandalwood are all useful as teas, tinctures or in freeze dried form.

Ayurvedic Formulas: Kidney Formula, Kaishore Guggulu.

Treatment for Kapha Urinary Problems
Food Plan: Kapha reducing diet.
Exercise: Kapha yoga poses, walking, weights, exercise machines, skiing, aerobics, bicycling.
Herbs: Uva Ursi, Echinacea, Goldenseal and Sandalwood are all useful. Additionally, it is important to avoid simple sugars, refined carbohydrates and full strength juice. To avoid becoming dehydrated, drink plenty of water. Foamy urine can be related to pancreatic problems.
Ayurvedic Formula: Sweet Ease.

Nervous System		
Vata Symptoms	*Pitta Symptoms*	*Kapha Symptoms*
Fear	Anger	Depression
Anxiety	Agitation	Emotional numbness
Insomnia	Judgmentalism	
Headache	Migraines	Dull headache
Shakiness		

Treatment for *Vata* Nervous System Problems
Food Plan: Vata reducing diet.
Exercise: Vata yoga poses, walking, weight, exercise machines, swimming.
Herbs: In general relaxants are good for *vata*. These include Lavender, Lemon Balm and Chamomile teas or oils along with Rose oil for massage and aromatherapy. Valerian, Scullcap and Passion Flower have been used for generations for stress and anxiety. Kava Kava is an effective relaxant that can be taken every 3 to 4 hours. We think of it as a "first aid" item to be taken as needed much as one takes aspirin. B-complex is also helpful for *vata, pitta* and *kapha*.
Ayurvedic Formulas: Triphala, Tranquil Mind

Treatment for *Pitta* Nervous System Problems
Food Plan: Pitta reducing diet.
Exercise: Pitta yoga poses, walking, weights, exercise machines, swimming.

Herbs: Aloe Vera and Sandalwood have a cooling effect on *pitta* imbalances as do the popular relaxants Chamomile, Lemon Balm and Rose. Kava Kava is also useful.
Ayurvedic Formulas: Liver Formula, Amalaki

Treatment for *Kapha* Nervous System Problems
Food Plan: Kapha reducing diet
Exercise: Kapha yoga poses, walking, weights, exercise machines, aerobics, running, bicycling, skiing.
Herbs: St. John's Wort and B-complex supplements are particularly good for depression.
Ayurvedic Formulas: Triphala, Mental Clarity

Summary

You have been presented with a variety of diagnostic tools to help you learn about your personal energy imbalances. In addition, you now have the needed dietary, exercise and herbal guidelines to help you reestablish balance. To reiterate, begin gradually and slowly. It is best to change diet and lifestyle habits slowly. Begin by cutting back the frequency and quantities of those foods which have the most serious impact on the *dosha* in question. Then begin substituting something else for old favorites most of the time. Occasionally you can splurge, but not too often if you wish to improve your *doshic* health, balancing *vata, pitta* and *kapha.*

If you do not exercise at present, quit making excuses and get your body moving in any way you can. Walking is good for starters. Anyone can start tasting herbal teas or using herbal essential oils. They are readily available in natural food stores or may be purchased through sources listed in a separate appendix. The least expensive way to taste is to purchase small quantities of bulk herbs. When you make a deep inner commitment to your state of health followed by self-diagnosis and modifications in your lifestyle along the lines we have suggested, you may be amazed at how much better you feel as your *doshas* become rebalanced.

CHAPTER 9

STAYING CLEAR OF TROUBLE: USING FOOD TO MAINTAIN BALANCE

IN CHAPTER SEVEN, food was discussed in terms of its qualities. The relationship between qualities, balance and health was emphasized. We suggested basic daily food selections and ways to move from convenience eating to more nutritious eating, and we provided food guidelines for a variety of health problems. In this chapter, food selection for prevention and optimal health is our focus, and we are more specific about the impact of various foods and nutrients. The major food groups needed by the body are discussed in detail. While there is some overlay, we think it is important to understand why particular foods are vital, regardless of what's happening in your *doshas*.

The first avenue of treatment is prevention. If you raise your awareness, use the tools presented in this book, and become conscious of imbalances before they develop into a disease, you will be in a position to maintain a healthier and longer life.

In this chapter we will:
- **Look at the importance of prevention in maintaining balance.**
- **Explore how food choices affect your state of balance.**

Prevention

The key to staying clear of trouble is a healthy immune system. The strength of your immunity depends on a number of things. First, the presence of toxins in your body begins to erode its strength. Second, imbalanced *doshas* impact its effectiveness. Third, if the digestive fire is out of balance, the body can't properly deal with the things it takes in. *Therefore, the strength of immunity depends on the state of toxins,* doshas *and digestive fire.* Although there are ways of treating the disease process at any stage, clearly the best way is to prevent it from developing in the first place. Nutrition, what you eat, plays an important role in strengthening or weakening your immune system. While the previous chapter focused on food and the *doshas*, in this chapter we will focus on the nutritional value of foods.

Through diet we ingest thousands of chemicals regularly that impact our immune system. However, everything we ingest—food, emotions, even thoughts—has an impact on our personal biorhythm, our individual way of interacting with the world. The body must "digest" everything it takes in. Even thoughts and emotions must be dealt with or they become crystallized and remain in the body. Everything held in the body that has not been properly metabolized creates stagnation, leading to accumulation of toxins and imbalance of the *doshas*.

How do you know when you are becoming imbalanced? Life is lived moment to moment and balance is maintained moment to moment. By being aware of your reaction to the food you had for dinner, to interactions with your spouse, children and friends, to the TV you watch, to the state of your spiritual being, you create an ongoing way of assessing and maintaining balance. Awareness of what is happening in the moment tells you where you are and where you're going. This state of awareness gives control, because awareness can lead to action. Dealing with imbalances at the very beginning, before they strengthen, is the key to prevention.

When you learned to ride a bicycle, in the beginning you flopped back and forth and perhaps took some tumbles from the bike. Now you maintain balance as you ride by gently adjusting your body weight from side to side. In the same way, you can learn to maintain the balance of your *doshas*. As you "ride" through life, if you are aware of little imbalances, which almost always exist, you can easily adjust. If the imbalances become bigger, you fall off the bike. To change the metaphor, the seed of disease begins in the moment. If the seed is not watered and cultivated, disease does not develop. The key is to become aware of the qualities affecting you.

In Chapter One, we talked about your basic constitution (and your individual DNA) as being your blueprint for life. The function of this blueprint is to support the body and tissues. This blueprint is your bull's eye for balance. Staying in that bull's eye requires that you become aware of what you are doing and how you are leading your life. You become what you experience in life. Whether or not you remain healthy depends on how you deal with your moment to moment existence. Every single experience is an instruction to behave in a certain way. This instruction is the preventive value of self-awareness, because it becomes moment to moment, not crisis to crisis or inspiration to desperation. If small imbalances are ignored, they become bigger and bigger. Like increases like. The best way to correct an imbalance is to use the opposite quality at every level—physically, emotionally, mentally and spiritually.

Nutrition: Food as Medicine

There is truth to the statement that we are what we eat, that our daily food choices are a keystone of maintaining balance and a healthy immunity. Over 2000 years ago Hippocrates said that food is our best medicine. This statement is as true for us today as it was then.

In this section, we tell you the ideal way to eat and why certain foods are ideal. Many people don't or can't eat this way, at least initially. In an appendix, we present common food patterns and suggest ways of easily including more nutrients. Going from "where you are" currently to where you eat for maximal health is a slow, gradual process. Begin with where you are. For example, if you now eat many of your meals at fast food restaurants, begin there and slowly improve your food selections.

How much should we eat each day? How much food we put into our bodies each day is certainly important and will vary with each individual. However, even more important is the right choice of food. A person can be over-nourished in calories and still be starved in nutrients. The high rate of obesity in America is proof of that fact. The human body will still be "hungry" as long as it is deficient in the necessary vitamins, minerals, fiber and other necessities. If you consume a diet rich in life-giving nutrients, you will be free of cravings and your appetite will be balanced. Too many people in our affluent country are "starving to death," in spite of obesity, because of a lack of proper nutrition. Too many lack the feelings of satisfaction and fulfillment that a nutrient rich diet provides.

So how much should you eat if your food choices are nutrient rich? If your diet consists of carefully chosen food and is free of "empty" calories, the amount needed is quite small. Diets of people around the world noted for longevity tend to be lower in calories than our standard American diet. The Vilcambayas of South America, the Hunzas of the Himalayas, as well as the long-lived people of Georgia in Russia, who are vigorous and active in their nineties and beyond their hundredth year, maintain an average consumption of 1500 to 1800 calories per day. In this country, we would consider that a weight loss diet. However, this amount of food is standard daily fare for these people. Calorie restriction in human beings appears to extend life and health.

Ongoing studies in animals since the 1950s have consistently produced results that confirm observations made of long-lived people around the world. Animals that are fed low calorie, nutrient rich diets live much longer than feed-at-will animals in control groups. The coats of low-calorie animals are shiny and without traces of gray, and they are resistant to disease. Studies indicate an increase of 20% to 50% in life expectancy.

Diet is certainly one of the major secrets for longevity. The opinion of many is that our preprogrammed genetic lifespan is 120 years. Roy Walford, MD, at UCLA, author of *The 120 Year Diet*,[1] has been conducting experiments with mice for the last 30 years. His studies support that a calorie restricted but nutrient rich diet increases longevity. However, lifespan without health span is meaningless. Health span indicates the amount of time in good health related to longevity. Animals in the wild maintain a health span until just before they die. In other words, they "live" until they die. Statistics show a greatly shortened health span in human beings. Another observation of long-lived people around the world is that they "live" until they die. It is increased quality of life, as well as length of life, that we want to promote through this book.

Let's be clear that when we speak about calorie restriction we do not mean malnutrition. Our approach utilizes a diet rich in all the necessary nutrients. The calories it deletes are empty calories, including refined sugar, breads made with refined flour, or excess alcohol. Our approach to diet, combined with appropriate lifestyle and exercise, helps maintain a strong immune system.

So What Should We Eat? When choosing your foods, eat as close to nature as possible and choose organically grown foods when they are available. Fresh organically grown food is nutrient rich and also contains the life force, so necessary for us to take in every day. Stay away from processed, frozen or canned foods, which are depleted of nutrients and the life force. In a nutshell, your daily diet should consist of fresh fruits and vegetables, adequate protein, some fat and high quality carbohydrates. Include five to seven servings a day of fresh fruits and vegetables. When choosing protein, be aware that eating too little will cause loss of muscle mass, including cardiac muscle, and eating too much protein will stress the kidneys. Too much and the wrong kind of fat will increase the probability of cancer and cardiovascular disease. Eating too little fat can also be harmful. The subject of carbohydrates is confusing. Many conflicting guidelines are in print. We discuss what kinds of carbohydrates are best for each constitution. We are best fed by the fiber and carbohydrates that naturally occur in fresh fruits and vegetables as well as in some whole grains. Let's look at each of these categories in more detail.

Vegetables. Vegetables head the list. In spite of all the conflicting information about protein, fats and carbohydrates, everyone agrees about the importance of eating a wide variety of vegetables. In the chapter on treatment, we were specific about which choices are best for *vata, pitta* or *kapha*. In this chapter, we speak more broadly. Look around and observe that many people do not eat any vegetables (other than french fries). This deficiency deprives them of needed nutrients for proper digestion and liver cleansing, and long term will most certainly lead to degenerative physical changes.

Green Leafy Vegetables. Dark green leafy vegetables offer an abundance of vitamins and minerals. Bitter greens such as kale, turnip greens, dandelion greens, etc., can be cooked and eaten, including the juices (called pot liquor in the South where Margaret grew up), and are a good source of many nutrients, including calcium and other minerals. *Eating dark green vegetables, including kale, is tied to lower rates of gastrointestinal, esophageal, stomach, lung, colon, oral and throat cancers and sometimes to cancers of all types.*

Some of these greens have a strong taste. A bit of sweetener, such as Stevia,[2] will cut the bitterness and make the greens more palatable. Remember that "bitter is better for the liver," and bitter greens help liver function. Other greens can be eaten raw in salads, but stay away from lifeless iceberg lettuce, which is lacking in nutrients.

Although cooking leafy greens destroys some of their nutrients, it makes other nutrients, such as beta carotene, more available for bodily use. It is wise to include both raw and cooked in our diets.[3]

Cruciferous Vegetables. In spite of George Bush's highly publicized dislike of broccoli, cruciferous vegetables, such as broccoli, brussels sprouts and cabbage, have been shown to have many health benefits, including anti-cancer action.

Broccoli appears to be a versatile cancer fighter. As a dark green vegetable, it emerges high in numerous lab tests designed to identify foods with cancer-counteracting potential. It also tops the food lists of people who have lower rates of all cancers, and, in particular, cancer of the esophagus, stomach, colon, lung, larynx, prostate, oral cavity and pharynx. As a member of the cruciferous family, broccoli ranks high against colon cancer. In fact, in some tests broccoli looks even better than its close cousin, cabbage, which is an acknowledged superstar in this area. Probably due to its abundance of chlorophyll, broccoli is extraordinarily potent in blocking cell mutations which precede cancer.

Brussels sprouts also boost the body's defenses. This vegetable, along with cabbage and broccoli, is included in the diets of people with low rates of cancer in general and colon and stomach cancer in particular. If you ask people around the world with low rates of cancer what they eat, green vegetables such as brussels sprouts are mentioned consistently.

Scientists have discovered specific chemicals in brussels sprouts that retard cancer in laboratory animals, including chlorophyll, indoles, dithiolthiones, carotenoids and glucosinolates. Animals that eat such foods or compounds and then are exposed to potent cancer causing chemicals are less likely to develop cancers than those fed no brussels sprouts or their active compounds.

Cabbage has an ancient and esteemed place in medical folklore. In ancient Rome, cabbage was regarded as a panacea. In modern times, modern folk medicine also hails cabbage as an anti-ulcer remedy. Cabbage, unquestionably, is one of the unassuming, unappreciated true stars of the food pharmacy. In studies to find the most potent anticancer foods for humans, cabbage regularly appears at the top. Cabbage's main claim to fame is its potential for preventing cancer.

Large population surveys in Greece, Japan and the United States link cabbage to protection against colon cancer.

What makes the cabbage connection so fascinating is that in the lab scientists can match and explain the human findings in chemical terms. In the 1970s Dr. Lee Wattenberg isolated chemicals from the cabbage family, called indoles, that block cancer formation in animals. He and others meticulously worked out precisely how these and other chemicals in cabbage suppress the activation of cancer-causing substances in animals. Cabbage and its cousins, brussels sprouts, broccoli and cauliflower, appear to guard cells against the very first onslaughts that may progress to full-fledged cancer.[4]

Scientific studies have also indicated that cabbage juice is beneficial in treating stomach ulcers. These studies generally agree that the cabbage's healing factors are present only when taken raw and usually as juice.[5]

Don't forget cabbage includes not only the typical head cabbage common in the United States, but also bok choy, a white stalk with green floppy leaves, and Chinese cabbage, an elongated bundle of leaves and core, as well as celery. All are of the cruciferous vegetable family that contains anticancer chemicals.

Eat at least some of your cabbage raw, unless your *vata* is excessive. Some therapeutic compounds are partly destroyed by heat. Some studies have found that raw cabbage (red as well as green) protects against stomach cancer.

Carrots. The most thrilling thing about carrots is their enormous promise in curtailing some of the most virulent, incurable cancers, notably of the lung and pancreas. Studies show that intake of modest amounts of carrots, and specifically the beta carotene in carrots, may retard cancer progression as well as disrupt the mechanism that first turns cells into growing malignancies.

With regularity, carrots turn up in studies pinpointing specific foods that ward off cancer. For example, a well-constructed 1986 Swedish study designated carrots as one of two prominent dietary barriers to pancreatic cancer. The other dietary barrier was citrus fruit.

The research tying vegetables and fruits containing beta carotene to less lung cancer is extensive. Additionally, high beta carotene foods have been linked to lower risk of cancers of the larynx, esophagus, prostate, bladder, cervix and, in a study among elderly people in Massachusetts, of all types of cancer. In lab studies, feeding carrots to rats blocked liver tumors.

Raw carrots decrease blood cholesterol. In one study, eating 200 grams of raw carrots (about two and a half medium size carrots) every morning for breakfast cut blood cholesterol an average of eleven percent. The carrots also increased the bulky weight of the stool by about twenty-five percent, which helps keep the colon healthy.

To get the most anticancer protection, eat at least some carrots cooked. Cooking releases carotenes, believed to be the active agents in shielding tissue against carcinogenic attacks. You get two to five times more carotene from cooked carrots than from raw ones. But don't overdo it; carrots cooked until they are mushy lose much of their precious carotene.[6]

Blended Soups. There are many vegetables to choose from, each with its own special health benefits. One easy and delicious way to incorporate vegetables into your diet is by making blended soups. Any vegetable can be steamed, perhaps with an added onion, a bit of garlic and some culinary herbs and seasonings, and then placed in a blender to make a smooth soup. If you dislike broccoli, this method is a delicious way to consume this vegetable and hardly realize what you are eating. Various greens, carrots or asparagus also make delicious soups. You don't even need to add milk or cream. Try a spoonful of nonfat plain yogurt on top of the soup. Delicious!

Buy organically grown vegetables, if at all possible. Not only will you avoid pesticide residue, you will also enjoy more flavor and higher nutritional value. Although organic foods may seem more expensive, compare the price you pay for them with the price you pay for processed food.

Fruits and Berries. Here is another category of foods about which there is little debate. The brightly colored substances found in fruits and berries are called flavonoids, which account for a significant percentage of the chemical constituents of these plants. Flavonoids, referred to as "biological response modifiers," possess anti-inflammatory, antiallergic, antiviral and anticarcinogenic properties. The potent antioxidant activity of flavonoids may be their most important healing aspect.

Flavonoids can be found in a wide variety of fruits, vegetables and many herbs. They are abundantly found in the white pulp of citrus fruits and in grapes, plums, black currants, apricots, buckwheat, cherries, blackberries, blueberries and rose hips.

Deeply Colored Berries. Deeply colored berries are more than just beautiful. They are good for you. Eat them in season and find an organic source. Each summer Margaret eagerly anticipates the wild blueberries in Maine. Freshly picked from an organic field, these berries contain many nutrients, including flavonoids, necessary for good health. Raspberries are also nutritious, as are cherries, blackberries and strawberries. If you have a good organic source, freeze or dry these berries and preserve them for later. Don't add sugar. They are naturally sweet.

Other Fruits. The old saying, "An apple a day keeps the doctor away," has a ring of truth. An apple contains many important nutrients, as well as fiber. In Greek mythology, apples were said to heal all ailments. In American folk medicine, the apple is called the king of fruits, a neutralizer of the body's excess acids. Modern scientific investigations find apples a versatile and potent package of natural drugs that deserve their reputation for keeping doctors away. The fruit helps keep the cardiovascular system healthy. Italian, Irish and French researchers have all confirmed that eating apples puts a dent in blood cholesterol.

The apple's secret drug is pectin, that soluble type of fiber that goes into jelly. Pure pectin extracted from fruits is a well known anticholesterol agent. But pectin alone does not explain the apple's powers, for a whole apple itself is a much more powerful cholesterol depressor than all the pectin squeezed out of it.

Apples are good for diabetics and others who want to avoid steep rises in blood sugar. Apples rank near the bottom of the "glycemic index" (a measurement of how fast blood sugar rises after eating particular foods). This means that despite an apple's natural sugar content, it does not spur a rapid rise in blood sugar. The fruit keeps the throttle on excess insulin, and as with other foods that do this, also lowers blood cholesterol and blood pressure.

Whole fresh apples may help ward off cancer, because they contain caffeic or chlorogenic acid, which blocks cancer formation in lab animals dosed with potent carcinogens. Be sure to eat an apple's skin; it is especially high in pectin fiber. Apple juice contains little pectin and cannot be expected to lower blood cholesterol, blood pressure or stabilize blood sugar. Apple juice also has much lower concentrations of anticancer chemicals.[7]

Bananas are also an important food, and they come in their own portable wrapper. They first emerged in the medical literature as a cure for ulcers in the early 1930s. More recent researchers have discovered that bananas work like the most sophisticated drugs. If you were designing an antiulcer drug, you would probably first look for one to neutralize or suppress the acid destroyers of the stomach lining. That's what common antiulcer drugs, such as antacids and cimetidine (Tagamet), do. Only one drug takes a different approach, carbenoxolone, infrequently used because it also induces high blood pressure. Nevertheless, it is an idea copied from nature, because its action is to increase the mucous lining of the stomach. Instead of knocking out the aggressors, it builds a better defensive wall.

In the same way, bananas strengthen the surface cells of the stomach, forming a sturdier barrier against noxious acids. However, bananas do not raise blood pressure. Researchers say bananas stimulate the proliferation of cells in the stomach lining, and also trigger the release of a protective layer of mucus that rapidly seals off the surface of the stomach lining, preventing excess hydrochloric acid and pepsin in the stomach from doing further damage. (In other words, bananas increase *kapha* in the cells of the stomach lining.) Bananas also contain potassium as well as an important kind of soluble fiber. Again, organic is better, if you can find a source.[8]

Without getting into detailed "rules" about what foods should be eaten with other foods, there is one bit of food combining information to take seriously when it comes to any fruit, melon and berry. Fruit is digested more rapidly in the stomach than other foods. If fruit arrives in the stomach alone, it is digested and moved out within an hour. However, if fruit is eaten with other foods—for example, banana with cereal and milk—the stomach becomes confused and doesn't know which food to tackle first. The result may be fermentation and a lack of proper digestion, often leading to discomfort due to the formation of toxins, resulting from insufficient digestion. Therefore, apply this "rule" and your stomach will thank you. Eat your fruits on an empty stomach or between meals.

A word about juices: When you drink the juice of any fruit or vegetable you are consuming a concentrated food. All of the fiber and solids have been taken out, removing the necessity for chewing. Because of this concentration, it is easy to consume a large amount quickly. Don't drink any juice too fast, as if you are consuming water. Sip slowly, savoring each mouthful, and perhaps dilute it a bit with filtered water. Eating a food close to the form in which nature provides is always preferable.

Fiber and Grains. This category opens up a bit more debate. Certainly there is no debate about the importance of staying away from refined grains, such as bread and baked goods made with bleached white flour. It is understood that the refinement process removes valuable nutrients. The subject of grains becomes cloudy when we talk about wheat. Many people are sensitive to the gluten in wheat. Wheat is a primary allergen. If you have problems with allergies, one of the first things to cut from your diet is wheat to see if there is an improvement of symptoms. (Another primary allergen is dairy.) There are many other grains from which to choose. Spelt, an ancient form of wheat, is being rediscovered, and spelt flour, cereals and breads are now available, especially in whole food stores. Other grains to investigate include millet and quinoa. Try these grains made into a pilaf with some chopped vegetables. The flavor of millet is strong and the texture is coarse. We are partial to quinoa.

Rice has long been available and most people can handle this grain. We use Indian basmati rice, because it is an easy to digest grain with a delightful aroma. Indian basmati is widely available in natural food stores and many supermarkets.

You might question the use of Indian basmati rice because it appears to be a refined white rice. However, there are a number of factors to take into consideration. Ayurvedic cooking seldom uses brown rice, because it is more difficult to digest. In addition, it is too heating for *pitta* and too heavy for *kapha*.

Basmati rice is parboiled, which retains many of its nutrients, in particular the B vitamins. Then it is aged for two years before it is used. The resulting rice is light and easy to digest. Parboiling places the nutrient value in between that of whole grain brown rice and refined white rice. The ease of digestion of Indian basmati makes it an excellent choice, especially for *vata* and *pitta*.

Another subject with conflicting views is fiber. Fibrous foods include fruits, vegetables and whole grains. Certainly we all need adequate fiber in our diets for the smooth movement of digestion through the colon. However, much of the fiber recommended today is separated from its whole food source—wheat bran, rice bran, etc. In our opinion, it is preferable to consume fiber with the whole food— whole grains, whole fruits and vegetables, etc., because it is preferable to eat as close to nature as possible. There are two types of fiber, soluble and insoluble. The bran in grains and the fibrous content of vegetables are insoluble fiber and pass through the digestive tract like a "broom." Bananas are an excellent source of soluble fiber.

Organic Meats and Fish. There is too much information available today for health conscious people to ignore the necessity of consuming organically grown poultry and meats whenever possible. Poultry and meats that have been commercially raised contain hormones and antibiotics. We just don't know the long term effects of these substances on our health. Increased consciousness is being raised around these issues. Fortunately, it is now possible to obtain organically raised poultry and meats in most locations. They are more expensive than non-organic but worth the price.

Fish is valuable in your diet, especially cold water fatty fish such as salmon, from which we receive high quality omega-3 oils. However, our polluted oceans are bringing the safety of consuming fish into question. In spite of the value of this food, we suggest caution. Be sure the fish you consume comes from clean waters. In addition, there are also unanswered questions about the safety and food value of farm raised fish, such as salmon. These fish are fed Purina Fish Chow and have no opportunity to eat the wild foods of the ocean. Perhaps a better source of essential omega-3s is flaxseed oil, a safe plant source.

An adequate supply of protein is essential for health. If you are a vegetarian, being sure you are eating enough protein is difficult, but not impossible. Vegetarians almost always need to take a supplement of B12 and Folic Acid. For those of us who are not vegetarians, about four ounces of lean, organically grown, high quality poultry or meat each day is an adequate amount. Too much is hard on the kidneys. However, if we consume too little, we may lose muscle mass.

What is too much or too little? It depends on the individual. However, we can certainly say that a person who regularly eats a 16 ounce steak, even if that person is quite a large man, is consuming too much protein. Excess protein creates an acid condition in the system, and an acid environment invites disease, especially inflammatory diseases, and strains the kidneys. The opposite extreme might be a person who never eats any form of animal protein, including eggs. This type of diet restriction may well lead to loss of muscle, including cardiac muscle. We recommend about four ounces of lean organic poultry, meat or fish each day.

Eggs. The much-maligned egg is now returning to its proper position of high esteem. Because of their rich nutrient content and easy digestibility, eggs are one of the best sources of bioavailable protein. Eggs contain all eight essential amino acids and are rich in essential fatty acids. The egg is a nearly perfect food and can be tolerated by most people, even those who are extremely ill. Cooked with care—soft boiled or gently scrambled—an egg is an extremely valuable addition to our diets.

The egg as an acceptable food was thrown out a number of years ago because of its cholesterol content. However, along with cholesterol, an egg contains the necessary nutrients to properly utilize the cholesterol. Cholesterol is a necessary component of a healthy body and, if we do not have enough in our systems, our bodies produce it to fill the need. What we need to be mindful of is a properly functioning liver, which produces cholesterol. A diseased liver will produce excess cholesterol even if the diet contains none.

If you have a tendency toward inflammatory conditions, you may wish to be moderate in egg consumption, because eggs are a bit high in some acids that can increase inflammation.

Choose only eggs from healthy chickens in a free-range environment, because they are free of hormones and pesticides. Eggs from these chickens have deeply colored yolks rich in omega-3 oils. Eggs of this quality can be safely added to a baby's diet. Compare these eggs to those from chickens cooped in a close environment and fed commercial foods containing antibiotics and hormones. The yolks of these commercially produced eggs are pale and nutrient deficient, in addition to containing residues of antibiotics and hormones from feed.

Milk. The first thing to be said about milk is that it is not the best source of calcium, because it is too high in protein and phosphorous, which reduce calcium utilization. Other sources, including the green leafy vegetables discussed above, are better sources of readily available calcium for the body.

Milk is appropriate for some people but not for others. As we mentioned above, if you have allergies, two of the major allergens are wheat and milk. Cut these foods from your diet first to see if there is improvement in your allergic reactions.

If you do drink milk, it should be consumed alone and not with other food, because it is a complex food. Consuming it with other foods makes digestion difficult. Cold milk is hard to digest and creates mucus. This can be avoided by boiling milk. Bringing a cup of milk to a boil and drinking it, especially at bedtime, is a relaxing drink. Adding half a teaspoon of Turmeric to this milk adds an immune boosting herb and creates a delicious deep yellow colored drink. We will discuss Turmeric in the next chapter.

Milk is another food that needs to be organic, and organically produced milk products are becoming widely available, even in supermarkets. The addition of growth hormone to the feed of cows raises questions about its effect on health. That hormone, along with antibiotics given to the cows and pesticides used in their food, are substances to be avoided if possible.

Goat's milk is becoming widely available. Because of the size of its fat molecule, this milk is more easily digested by human beings. Many babies and young children who cannot tolerate cow's milk can easily digest goat's milk.

Ghee (Clarified Butter). *Ghee* is highly prized by Ayurveda. It is one of the few fats that does not break down when heated (perhaps the only one). We use it almost exclusively for any type of sautéing or stir-frying.

In addition to its value in cooking, *ghee* is an esteemed medicine in Ayurveda. It is frequently used as a carrier for various herbs. According to Ayurveda, the older the *ghee*, the more medicinal its properties. According to Ayurveda, *ghee* will not raise your cholesterol, because the removal of milk solids in *ghee* removes most of the cholesterol. However, use it sparingly. One teaspoon at each meal added to your food is an appropriate amount.

Because pesticides, hormones and antibiotics are absorbed in fat, it is quite important to choose organically produced unsalted butter to make *ghee*. If you want to make your own *ghee*, follow the boxed recipe.

Ghee (Clarified Butter)

Place one pound of unsalted butter (be sure to use unsalted) in a heavy, medium-sized pan. Turn on the heat to medium until butter melts. (Choose a time when you are close by to watch.)

Turn down the heat until the butter just boils and continue to cook at this heat.

Do not cover the pot. The butter will foam and sputter and then begin to quiet down.

In about 15 minutes, the butter will begin to smell like popcorn and turn a lovely golden color. Whitish curds will begin to form on the bottom of the pot. When these whitish curds turn a light tan color, the *ghee* (butter) is ready. Take it off the heat immediately, because it burns easily at this stage.

Let the *ghee* cool slightly. Pour the *ghee* through a fine sieve and store in a glass container with a tight lid. Discard the curds caught in the sieve.

Ghee can be kept covered on the kitchen shelf and requires no refrigeration. It will keep indefinitely as long as no wet or dirty spoon is used to dip from the container. Moisture will create conditions for bacteria to grow and spoil the *ghee*.[9]

Yogurt. Many of the long-lived people mentioned above include yogurt in their diets. There are many health benefits to yogurt, including the maintenance of healthy bacteria in the colon. Yogurt is a digestive aid and we frequently end a meal with *lassi*, a drink made from yogurt. Try this delicious drink to end your meal instead of a sweet dessert. For those with slow metabolism or high acidity, a drink made from yogurt can be helpful. Here is a recipe we use.

Lassi

Place one cup of plain non-fat yogurt in a blender.

Add one cup of water.

Although there are many variations, we like a bit of vanilla and some kind of sweetener (perhaps a few drops of Stevia) added to the above.

Blend until smooth.

Pour into glasses.

Top with roasted ground cumin seeds.[10]

Good quality yogurt is available in supermarkets and natural food stores. If possible, choose organic and nonfat with acidophilus and without artificial flavors and preservatives.

Mushrooms. When we say "mushroom," we think of those white button vegetables in the supermarket. However, the world of mushrooms is vast and a marvelous medicinal storehouse all to itself. Medicinal mushrooms make a significant contribution to the healing process by enhancing and stimulating the body's own immune system. They are being used today to treat diseases such as cancer and AIDS. Let's look at a few representatives from this magical kingdom.

*Shiitake (**Lentinus edodes**).* We have all had the experience of eating those black mushrooms included in many Chinese dishes. However, few of us have incorporated them into our home food preparation. These mushrooms are delicious and are packed with nutrients that boost immunity. Shiitake mushrooms have been the subject of many studies since they were discovered to possess choles-terol lowering properties. Because of their antitumor activity, they also inhibit the growth of cancer cells.

These mushrooms are widely available at this point, both fresh and dried. They can be expensive, so shop around. If you have access to a Chinese market, the price of dried shiitakes is quite reasonable. Just soak these dried mushrooms in hot water until they become soft and slice them to include in soup or a sitir-fry. Don't use the stems of this mushroom. Although they are not poisonous, if you consume too many, they may create nausea.

Reishi (*Ganodermum lucidum*). The reishi mushroom is not one we would want to include in our stir-fry, because it is hard and woody. However, the medicinal qualities of this plant are enormous. Reishi has a large range of therapeutic uses and can be found growing around the world. It can be taken as a powder or in a capsule.

Reishi is the perfect remedy for the typical American suffering from stress, who has depressed life force and is likely to be both deficient and toxic. Reishi is beneficial to the restoration of balance. It enhances immune function and improves both energy and sleep. It is used in cancer treatment to inhibit tumor growth.

Its actions will calm the nervous system and reduce insomnia, in addition to affecting the circulatory system by lowering blood pressure and blood cholesterol. This herb is considered a longevity tonic because of its antioxidant effect. According to Terry Williard, a well known herbalist, reishi's antimicrobial action works against bacteria, fungi and viruses. Several countries use this mushroom to treat cancer, AIDS, fibromyalgia and chronic fatigue syndrome. Look for reishi supple-ments in a natural foods store.

Maitake. The maitake mushroom is a prized medicinal mushroom from Japan. Its strongest effects are on the immune system. Unlike reishi, maitake is an edible mushroom. Dr. Williard also states that maitake has been used in treating AIDS and has been successful in reducing symptoms and slowing the progression of this disease. As an anti-cancer agent it has reduced tumors as well as the side effects of chemotherapy. It has also been shown to reduce blood pressure, help recovery from hepatitis and reduce blood sugar in diabetics. As a weight management herb, it produces slow but consistent results in weight loss.[11]

Medicinal mushrooms are powerful substances. The information included here is brief and has been included only to raise your awareness about these plants.[12]

Seaweeds. Do you know how healthful seaweeds are? Seaweeds, yuck! Those slimy things on the beach! Let's back off and take a look.

The powers of sea vegetables have been drawn upon for thousands of years for their ability to prolong life and prevent disease. The sea is the source from which all things arise and to which they return. The human body begins its development in a saline solution in the womb and is nourished and cleansed by blood that has almost the same composition as sea water.[13]

Sea plants contain as much as 10 to 20 times the minerals of land plants and an abundance of vitamins and other elements necessary for human metabolism, making them an excellent source for food and medicine. They are high in protein, as well as many minerals—calcium, iron, sodium, zinc and iodine. They also contain appreciable amounts of vitamins A, C and B-complex, including B-12. Seaweeds are known to aid the healthy growth of nails, hair, bones and teeth. They reduce blood cholesterol, aid digestion and keep the endocrine glands, especially the thyroid, functioning well. The sodium alginate in sea vegetables appears to neutralize radioactive substances in the body by binding to them and then harmlessly excreting them.[14]

There are a number of sea plants that are used in cooking and for medicinal purposes, including kelp, arame, dulse, hijiki. If you have been to a Japanese restaurant, perhaps you have had sushi wrapped in sheets of nori, another sea vegetable. We encourage you to include small quantities of sea vegetables in your diet, because of the rich source of trace minerals. A company called Maine Coast Sea Vegetables, located far north up the coast of Maine, has a number of products available. An easy way to include a daily dose of seaweed in your diet is to sprinkle a bit of their dried seaweeds on your food. A tiny pinch on your food each day is all you need.

Nuts and Seeds. Nuts and seeds got a bad name along with oils and fats in recent years, because they are high in calories. However, these little bundles of nutrition need to be reconsidered. They are excellent sources of protein and minerals, including calcium. Sunflower, pumpkin, sesame seeds and almonds are excellent choices. Be sure they are fresh and keep them refrigerated. Because of their high oil content, seeds easily become rancid, if not refrigerated. If they taste or smell somewhat "off," don't eat them, because rancid oil is toxic to the system. Nuts and seeds are best eaten raw and without salt. Roasting the nuts changes the quality of the oil. Peanuts, a legume and not a nut, should never be eaten raw, because of bacterial and fungal growth.

The Missing Ingredient? There is something more. So far we have been analytical about what each food contains in terms of nutrients and what it can do for us. But there is more to add to the total picture. Ayurveda speaks of *prana*, the vital life force. How do we receive this most vital life sustaining energy?

Nutrition, the food we eat, nourishes us on the level of the body. However, as food is digested and metabolized, it becomes much more than bodily nourishment. Because of the interrelatedness of our total being—body, mind and consciousness—the food we eat is transformed at the cellular level into something far beyond the physical, fueling both our energy supply and our level of awareness.

Dr. K. L. Chopra, a Hindu cardiologist and father of Dr. Deepak Chopra, said: "*Prana* is the vital life force of the universe, the cosmic force . . . and it goes into you, into me, with food. When you cook with love, you transfer the love into the food and it is metabolized."[15]

Deborah Kesten, in her book *Feeding the Body, Nourishing the Soul*, tells how there is more to food than the biological effects it has on the body. She tells of discovering that "all of life is interconnected: the sun, wind and rain that 'fertilizes' food; the soil, plants and food animals; the many hands who grow and harvest our food; those who bring it to our local grocer; cooks who prepare it; and the family and friends with whom we share our food. In a profound way, we are all in relationship to food and with each other."[16] Food is more than simply nourishment for the body. It becomes a potent metaphor for relationship to consciousness and social relationships. It is no accident that almost all successful social events include food, or that people routinely gather around food. Eating together nourishes our bodies, our social interactions and our consciousness. Bringing a loving and meditative awareness to food becomes a vehicle for connecting to Mother Nature, the Divine, the mystery that is life itself. We are one—body, mind and consciousness—and nourishment of consciousness, our spiritual essence, is essential to health.

The current biologically oriented nutrition paradigm has given us much useful information. However, it presents an incomplete picture. One of the purposes of this book is to expand consciousness and help formulate a new paradigm around health for the new millennium. We need an understanding of spiritual nourishment as a part of a new nutritional paradigm.

Pitta is responsible for transformation. Dr. Lad, our Ayurvedic teacher, speaks about the transformation of an apple into the cells of the body. "There is an apple hanging in the tree. That apple is outside of your body. You pluck the apple and start chewing. The *pitta* in the stomach digests the apple. The pectin part of the apple is sent to the colon to bind the stool. The sugar part of the apple goes with the blood into the muscles, bones and even into the reproductive tissue. The transformation of the apple into blood glucose is governed by *pitta*. When you eat food, that food undergoes the process of digestion, absorption and assimilation and then the food becomes a part of the cells. But the moment water, food and air molecules enter the cell, they become intelligence. Finally, *pitta* transforms food into pure consciousness."[17]

Raising awareness around our food choices acknowledges the inherent sacred quality of food: that it is life-filled and life-giving, offering biological, psychological and spiritual sustenance. When we eat, the awareness we bring to our food needs to include more than the nutrients we are consuming.

Oprah Winfrey puts it in a plain and beautiful way when she talks about observing some beautiful fruit: "I was looking at the fruit in the basket and I started to feel the fruit kind of giving itself up to the world. . . . I could feel the essence of the fruit. I swear to you, I could. And I had to stop myself from crying from looking at the fruit . . . I was so grateful for the little pomegranates and their seeds."[18]

As we raise our awareness and experience the connection of food with more than the physical, along with absorbing food's nutrients comes the possibility of integrating the consciousness of all who have had contact with the food, including our own. In this way, the food we eat may help us to stumble across our true essence: the unity and oneness of all life suggested by saints, mystics and scientists alike. Through this awareness, this consciousness, we welcome the vital essence of life into our total being—body, mind and consciousness.

CHAPTER 10

Protecting Yourself from Toxins in Your Food

In this section we discuss many common foods that have a negative impact on health. These common items that we all "know" are "bad" for us are "bad" primarily because of excessive consumption. Alternatives are available, and we will suggest many. So, as you read, don't be overwhelmed by all the negative effects we are about to identify.

Life is much more complex as we begin a new millennium, and the quality of our food supply raises many questions. In particular, we are concerned about toxins in our food, because we don't know how the chemicals, antibiotics and growth hormones increasingly being introduced into our food supply by modern agriculture are affecting our bodies. A number of health hazards are inherent in common foods and drinks. You might be tempted to think that "nothing" can be enjoyed and feel overwhelmed or hopeless. While it is true that our air, water and food are polluted, there is much we can do to strengthen our immune systems in order to maintain a state of balance. We will share with you some ideas of how to make changes slowly, at your own pace, starting with where you are at the moment.

Toxins in Food

Each of the approximately 3,000 different chemicals currently used in agriculture has been tested for toxicity in animals. However, each has been tested in isolation, one chemical at a time, and for only a few weeks or months, before being released into the marketplace. Unfortunately, these chemicals have not been tested in conjunction with each other.

We don't know their combined effects, short term or long term. We are guinea pigs for the chemical companies.

Artificial chemicals are foreign to our bodies and may have a tremendous impact on the immune system. The point is we do not know. We are just beginning to learn. Most agricultural chemicals have been manufactured from petrochemicals and are highly *pitta* producing. In addition the ability of our bodies to process them is questionable. Much of the time they get stored in the fat cells of our bodies, because there is no adequate exit route and our bodies can't successfully eliminate them. Many are in such an alien form that our liver can't handle them. As they travel through the bloodstream and lymphatic system, our immune system recognizes them as foreign substances. It struggles to neutralize them but often fails, so they are stored in our tissues as toxins and build up over the years, eventually eroding our health.[1] In addition, the consumption of antibiotics in our food chain results in resistance of our bodies to antibiotics when we need them to fight disease.[2]

A number of recent newspaper articles raise troubling questions about our food supply. *The Arizona Republic* reported on a study indicating pesticides may cause brain damage in young children. The study revealed that exposure to pesticides in the womb or at an early age may cause permanent brain defects that may be exacting a toll on the intelligence, motor skills and personalities of infants, toddlers and preschoolers.[3] The study went on to suggest there may be a correlation between pesticide use and hyperactivity in children.

Bacteria resistant to the most powerful antibiotics used to treat infections in people have been found in chicken feed. "Finding such organisms on the threshold of the human food supply is an ominous sign."[4] One is reminded of the animal feed problem leading to Mad Cow Disease, which continues to receive so much publicity. This neurological disorder in cows was caused by the contamination of their food by adding diseased animal products to it. The problem surfaced in Great Britain. Although no direct connection was made to that specific disorder being passed on to humans by consumption of the diseased meat, suspicions were roused and many cattle were slaughtered in an effort to bring the problem under control. The disease has resurfaced in France and other European countries. In addition, the disease has now been identified in humans. Two people in France and 80 in Britain have died from its human form, and 89 people across Europe have been infected.[5]

To compound the issue of food safety, *The New York Times* published a front page article, just days before this section was written, titled "Farmers' Right to Sue Grows, Raising Debate on Food Safety."[6] The article reports that ever since apple sales plummeted a decade ago, due to publicity by CBS News about the toxic effects of the chemical Alar, used by many apple growers, food producers have been fighting back. At this point, 13 states have passed laws to help protect farmers and food companies from criticism that could lead consumers to shun their products. The article noted that one such law was used by the group of Texas cattlemen who sought damages from Oprah Winfrey, the talk show host, after she made disparaging remarks on her show about beef. According to the article, the laws are putting a chill on the continuing debate about what we should eat. Food producers say they need protection against irresponsible claims, but critics say the laws cut off debate on evolving health issues. The article quotes a Seattle lawyer representing CBS in the apple suit: "It's like the Catholic Church telling Galileo in the 1620s that he was not allowed to trumpet a new viewpoint. . . . These laws are designed to lock orthodoxy in place. . . . If society wants to continue to have safe food, you need to have free and open discussion of the risks."

Ohio passed a food libel law in 1996. Because of this law, according to the above article, some people who have spoken out on food issues in the past say they now hesitate. "When I give speeches, I look around and think, Does someone have a tape recorder?" said a nurse and volunteer at the Ohio Sierra Club who speaks to groups about genetically engineered food. "I'm even afraid to say, 'This might be unsafe,'" she said, "because I'm fearful I could get sued." Despite intimidation tactics, the genetic engineering debate has grown.

And that's not all. *The New York Times* reported a recent food scare in Belgium.[7] "The entire nation is wondering what to eat these days after those foods (steak, chicken, eggs) were pulled from supermarket shelves or considered too suspect to eat because of cancer causing dioxin (a pesticide) feared to have spread through the Belgian food chain due to contaminated animal feed."

So how safe is our food chain? We don't really know and that is the problem. It is frightening to realize that profits for the food industry are more important than the safety of the people consuming its products.

Some of the chemicals widely used for agriculture in this country for many years—for example, DDT—are now outlawed in the United States, because they are dangerous to the food chain. However, this country continues to ship these chemicals to other countries. If we buy produce grown in Mexico, much of which is available in our super-markets, it may have been treated with these chemicals.

The only way we can eliminate toxic chemicals from our food is to choose to buy organic and/or to grow our own food. Organically grown food is becoming widely available throughout the United States. However, it is more expensive. Growing some of our own vegetables is possible for those of us with garden space, but is difficult or impossible for most of us today.

Organically grown food is our best choice. But if it is not available, choose fresh fruits and vegetables from your supermarket. The next best choice is frozen. Then comes processed food. At the bottom of the list is food that has been canned, because the canning process uses high heat which destroys most nutrients. However, it is better to use canned fruits and vegetables than no fruits and vegetables at all. The farther down the list you go, the fewer the nutrients and the presence of *prana*, the life force. It should be noted that processed and canned foods usually contain high quantities of salt and sugar to cover up a lack of flavor. Be sure to read the labels and make the best choices available.

Negative Nutrients: Coffee, Alcohol, Sugar and Salt

Negative nutrients are foods that remove more from the body than they put in. These substances draw down the vitamins and minerals already present in the body as the body attempts to process and eliminate them. Some of these substances are obvious, such as coffee and alcohol. But do you know how harmful sugar is to our bodies? And how about refined table salt?

Coffee. A strong relationship exists between drinking six or more cups of coffee a day and high cholesterol. High coffee consumption is also related to heart disease.[8] In addition, there is evidence supporting an association between consumption of caffeine and fibrocystic breast disease. Caffeine is known to stimulate overproduction of fibrous tissue and cyst fluid, which can lead to fibrocystic formations.[9] If you have fibrocystic breasts, the first line of treatment is to eliminate caffeine. Or, in accord with our emphasis on prevention, cut back on or eliminate coffee from your diet before fibrocystic changes begin.

Coffee consumption may contribute to elevated blood pressure readings. Although the effects of long-term caffeine consumption on blood pressure have not yet been clearly determined, one large study (6,321 adults) demonstrated a small but statistically significant elevation in blood pressure when comparing those who drank five or more cups a day to non-coffee drinkers.[10] Excessive coffee and other drinks containing caffeine may also cause symptoms of bowel upset. It should be noted that coffee increases *pitta* and creates an acidic condition in the body, leading to the leaching of calcium from the bones. Although the taste of coffee is bitter, an essential taste that needs to be included in the diet, there are better sources. For example, include bitter greens in your salad or as a cooked vegetable.

Should everyone eliminate coffee? Many people can drink one or two cups in the morning without apparent ill effects. If the caffeine doesn't interfere with your sleep, or if you don't have any of the conditions mentioned above, two cups a day probably does you no significant harm. However, we strongly urge cutting back if you are drinking more than two cups a day. If you continue to drink one or two cups, add a pinch of cardamom and ginger powder to the coffee to help protect your liver from the harmful effects of the caffeine. Coffee takes more from the body than it gives. If you have a compromised immune system in any way, stay away from coffee, colas and chocolate, all of which contain caffeine. Wean yourself from caffeine slowly, by adding more and more decaf each day. Then when totally on decaf, begin to eliminate coffee completely and switch to tea, a much better choice. A word about decaf: water processed decaf available in natural food stores is a better choice than the decaf available in supermarkets, beause it uses fewer harmful chemicals in the decaf process.

Alcohol. Chronic alcohol consumption can produce hypertension in some people, because it increases adrenaline secretion.[11] Alcohol ingestion suppresses the immune system, even in nutritionally normal people. Alcohol increases susceptibility to infections in animals, and alcoholics are known to be more susceptible to pneumonia.[12] Alcohol ingestion elevates cholesterol, triglycerides and uric acid levels, and increases the risk of atherosclerosis.[13] It is also known to disrupt normal sleep patterns.[14]

Alcohol may precipitate migraine headaches in some people. It causes constriction of the blood vessels.[15] Alcohol increases the absorption of toxins from the gut, along with impairing liver function. Because of this action, alcohol consumption is known to worsen psoriasis, because it increases *pitta*.[16] In addition, alcohol dehydrates the body by drawing water from the tissues.

Considering all of this negative information, is there anything positive to say about alcohol? Moderation is the key to everything. There has been considerable press about the benefits of red wine in preventing heart disease. In addition, many people find that a glass of wine with dinner helps with relaxation and a sense of well-being. In Eastern medicine, medicinal herbal wines are helpful in treating many conditions. Again, the key is moderation and proper usage.

Sugar. Sugar is a classic example of a negative nutrient and is dangerous for a variety of reasons. Sugar abuse results in low nutrient density; disruption of stable energy, pancreatic stress, adrenal stress, liver stress; cultivation of yeast overgrowth; undermining of immune competence.[17] Sugar is a good fuel for the body. If you are running a marathon, it is handy to have a bottle of Gatorade around, which is mostly sugar, some salt and a bunch of additives and food colorings. It will pump you up quickly. But in order to use the sugar to form energy in the body, you need vitamins and minerals not present in the sugar. If you are consuming a nutrient deficient diet, these vitamins and minerals will come out of muscle tissue and later on out of bone tissue. Eating a high sugar diet is a good way to predispose yourself to osteoporosis, because sugar acidifies the blood, causing the body to pull calcium out of your bones to neutralize the acid.

Sugar strongly impacts the immune system. If you eat four ounces (half a cup) of refined table sugar at one sitting, it may reduce your white blood cell activity by 50 percent for six hours, because sugar suppresses the activity of white blood cells. Your response might be that you would never eat that much sugar. However, examine carefully all the foods you eat. If you drink coffee, do you add sugar? How much? Is your meal composed of some processed food? If so, look at the label for the amount of sugar it contains. Do you eat desserts? How much sugar do they contain? A hundred years ago the so-called civilized Western world ate approximately five pounds of sugar per person per year. This sugar was unrefined, thick and dark. Currently in North America each person eats an average of 138 pounds of refined sugar per year.[18] Unrefined sugar contains some nutrients. However, all nutrients have been stripped from the refined white sugar so heavily consumed today.

We are losing the battle with obesity in part because of our consumption of sugar. Since fat was named the "Bad Guy" back in the 1970s, we have been consuming large amounts of fat free but sugar laden foods. During the last decade, Americans have reduced their fat intake at least two percent, but we have become 30 percent more overweight in almost the same time.[19] The right kind of fat is an essential nutrient that our bodies need. Sugar, on the other hand, is something we don't need at all, yet, on the average, Americans consume approximately their body weight in sugar each year.

Refined sugar acts more like a drug from which our bodies need to detoxify than a food. With many calories but no nutrients, sugar is one of the major causes (along with excess oil and salt) of America's weight problem and lack of good nutrition.

The dramatic increase in the consumption of refined sugar over the last one hundred years is a cause for great concern. Our bodies aren't programmed to handle this increase. The human body has not essentially changed since the Stone Age, yet we are ingesting many refined foods today that our bodies can't deal with. As a consequence, our bodies are developing a number of health problems related to modern culture, including weakened immunity, heart disease, high blood pressure, cancer and more. Today we are seeing an increase in the amount of adult onset diabetes, which didn't exist before the advent of refined white sugar and which still doesn't exist in some cultures where refined sugar consumption is low.

To help you get a better perspective on how concentrated refined sugar is, let's look at some statistics.[20] How many of you have eaten sugarcane? It is fibrous and takes a long time to chew. If you were to take 16 inches of a one-inch diameter stalk and refine it, the sugarcane would yield one teaspoon of refined sugar. Table sugar is the end-product of the refining of sugarcane. It is easy to eat one teaspoon of sugar, but it takes considerable time to chew through the 16 inches of sugarcane. In addition, sugarcane juice contains vitamins and minerals, which are removed in the process of refining.

Another illustration: A 15 ounce can of regular Coke contains 13 teaspoons of sugar. How many feet of sugarcane is that? You can down a can of Coke in 10 minutes. Small children consume Coke and then climb the walls because of hyperactivity caused by the sugar. To counteract that hyperactivity, they are then put on Ritalin so they can sit still.

If you have immune dysfunction, sugar is perhaps the most impor-tant item to remove from your diet. As we mentioned earlier in this section, the germ killing ability of white blood cells is slowed after consumption of sugar. Sugar creates an acid environment in the body, which sets up the possibility for the development of disease. Sugar interferes with the body's utilization of vitamin C, an important nutri-ent for immunity, and causes mineral imbalances and possible allergic reactions. In addition, it neutralizes the action of essential fatty acids, which we will discuss in the next section.

Our culture has become "sugarized" and expects an abundance of the sweet taste. Refined sugar should not be a component of the balanced diet. Evidence against sugar continues to mount. Even the recently developed Food Guide Pyramid warns Americans to limit their sugar consumption.

Other Sweeteners. If your diet contains large amounts of sugar, begin to cut back gradually. Doing anything "cold turkey" rarely works. First of all, substitute some natural sweeteners in place of refined sugar. Small amounts of maple syrup, molasses or honey are certainly better than refined sugar, because they contain micronutri-ents. However, your ultimate goal should be to reduce the total amount of sugars you consume, not simply to exchange white sugar for a more natural sweetener. The sweet taste is essential in the diet. However, the best way to satisfy the need for it is through fruits and other foods naturally high in this taste. We need to learn to enjoy the taste of foods as they are without any added sugar. This may take time, but it is worth the effort.

What about artificial sweeteners? They may seem like an easy way out, but these sweeteners can cause harm. The use of artificial sweeteners hasn't diminished Americans' sugar intake but seems to have given users more of a sweet tooth. In addition, artificial sweeteners haven't helped with weight.

Aspartame (Equal or NutraSweet) may deplete the body's supplies of chromium, a trace mineral important in sugar metabolism. Insufficient chromium leads to insulin inefficiency, which, in turn, leads to insulin resistance or carbohydrate intolerance. Aspartame can increase sugar and carbohydrate cravings, because the chemical phenylalanine, one of aspartame's components, blocks production of serotonin in the brain, which results among other things in more sugar and carbohydrate cravings and increases the likelihood of binge eating.[21]

And that isn't all. There is evidence that the use of aspartame destroys neurons and contributes to the development of brain and nervous system disorders, such as Alzheimer's disease.[22] Consumption of aspartame may also create neurological symptoms mimicking multiple sclerosis, lupus and Parkinson's. When the temperature of aspartame exceeds 80 degrees Fahrenheit, the wood alcohol in aspartame converts to formaldehyde and then to formic acid, which in turn causes metabolic acidosis, raising *pitta* in the body. This toxicity mimics neurological disorders. In many cases, neurological symptoms disappear if aspartame consumption is discontinued.[23]

Saccharin is also dangerous and has been suspected of causing cancer. In spite of the fact that saccharin has just been removed by the FDA from the list of unacceptable substances, we still advise caution. Don't use artificial sweeteners. They may be as harmful to your body as the sugar you are trying to replace. If you want to stay away from the calories in sugar, try Stevia.

Stevia. Both of us like Stevia, and we have found it a satisfying alternative to sugar and other sweeteners, because it does not raise blood sugar levels. *Stevia rebaudiana* (its botanical name) is a small shrub native to portions of Northeastern Paraguay and adjacent sections of Brazil. At present it is cultivated in many other countries, and its usage is rapidly growing. A powdered extract of Stevia has 30 times the sweetness of sugar, negligible calories, and does not raise blood sugar like other caloric sweeteners. The herb is available in many health food stores as a dietary supplement.

Stevia has been used for hundreds of years as a sweetener in South America and is currently widely used in Japan. When the Japanese government banned certain artificial sweeteners due to health concerns in the late sixties, the use of Stevia as a natural alternative increased dramatically. Its usage in Japan has also increased, because of increasing awareness of the detrimental effects of sugar and its contribution to such health problems as dental cavities, obesity and diabetes.

While Stevia has primarily been used as a sweetener in other parts of the world, it has also been investigated as an aid in regulating blood sugar metabolism, as an anti-hypertensive agent and as an anti-bacterial substance. Research is still preliminary, but several studies indicate some normalizing effects on the cardiovascular system, kidney function and blood pressure. As an herb, it is also used to treat imbalances of the pancreas.

Why has the use of Stevia been blocked for so long in the United States? One wonders if it has anything to do with lobbying on the part of the artificial sweetener industry. As of the writing of this book, the FDA allows Stevia to be imported only as a dietary supplement and has not yet put it on the GRAS (generally recognized as safe) list. The FDA's stance appears to be a compromise and to have political over-tones.

Is Stevia safe? A number of scientific studies have verified that its use is non-toxic, both short-term and long-term.[24] The rest of the world agrees and, in spite of the current controversy over it in the United States, Stevia is available, albeit on a qualified basis.

Salt. Sodium is essential to life. It plays countless roles in the body and without it we would cease to exist. However, sodium, as well as fat, is misunderstood. Both are nutrients we need for health, but not all forms are healthy. Just as there are "good" fats and "bad" fats, there are also "good" sources of sodium and "bad" sources.

We in this country consume far too much refined salt. The intake of the average American is two to three tablespoons a day, which equals

4,000 to 6,000 milligrams, double the FDA's maximum recommended daily quantity of 2,400 milligrams. No other mammal eats this much salt and no other mammal has the salt related health problems we do. High blood pressure was never seen in animals until researchers found they could induce it by adding large amounts of salt to their diets.[25]

Common table salt is a form of sodium that should be eliminated from our diets, because it does not properly excrete from our bodies. During the refining process, such salt is stripped of more than 60 trace minerals, leaving only sodium chloride. It is heated at such high temperatures that the chemical structure of the salt changes. Then it is chemically cleaned, bleached and treated with anticaking agents which prevent the salt from absorbing moisture. Because of these anticaking agents, refined salt does not dissolve and combine with the water and fluids present in our bodies. Instead, it builds up and leaves deposits in organs and tissues, causing severe health problems.

The two most common anticaking agents used are sodium alumino-silicate and alumino-calcium silicate. Both of these chemicals are sources of aluminum, which many believe is implicated in the development of Alzheimer's. The aluminum used in the refining process leaves a bitter taste in the salt, so sugar is added to hide the taste of the aluminum.[26] The above process produces a product that is hazardous to human health. Refined table salt should be avoided.

A source of sodium of which few of us are aware is salt softened water. The American Heart Association now warns that salt softened water can cause elevated sodium levels when drunk. However, bathing in this water can also increase sodium levels. Our skin is porous and absorbs whatever is put on it.

What are some of the diseases associated with consumption of excess salt?

• *Hypertension*. A person is said to have hypertension if there are consistent blood pressure readings above 140/90. This condition affects one in four adults and is one of the most common medical problems in the United States today.[27] High blood pressure is rare in countries where the diet is low in sodium.

Recent research shows that obtaining adequate potassium, magnesium and calcium may be as significant for high blood pressure prevention and control as lowering the intake of salt. The typical American diet is as *high* in sodium as it is *low* in these nutrients.[28] The ratio of these important nutrients is setting our bodies up for severe problems.

• *Osteoporosis.* Excess dietary sodium also increases the risk for osteoporosis and probably also kidney stones. Excess sodium in the tissues leads to calcium loss through the urine. Then the blood level of calcium falls, leading to withdrawal of calcium from the bones.

• *Stomach Ulcers and Stomach Cancer.* The stomach is particularly sensitive to refined salt. There is a strong correlation between the incidence of gastric ulcers and the consumption of refined salt. High intake of salt preserved, smoked and cured foods is a known risk factor for stomach and esophageal cancer. Sodium nitrites and nitrates in these foods can form nitrosamines in the stomach, some of the most potent cancer causing agents known. It is interesting to note that the Japanese, who have the highest incidence of stomach ulcers and stomach cancer in the world, consume more salt, nitrite and nitrate treated foods than any other culture.[29]

How much sodium each of us needs depends on who we are. The answer to our individual sodium requirements isn't as simple as many would like us to believe. While sodium needs do vary, reducing sodium too much can be just as harmful as consuming large amounts of it. Too little sodium can cause spasms, poor heart rhythm and even sudden death. Low salt, not no salt, appears to be best as a permanent way of eating for most of us.[30] However, all of us can benefit from removing refined salt from our diets.

Monosodium Glutamate (MSG) is another form of sodium we should avoid. Recent scientific studies suggest that long term ingestion of substances such as MSG contribute to the development of diseases of both the brain and nervous system. We have already discussed the effects of aspartame on the body, and MSG is included in this same category of possible damage to the brain and nervous system.[31] Many processed foods contain MSG. If you use any of these foods, read the labels carefully.

What kind of salt is acceptable?

• *Sea Salt.* Commercial sea salt is better than refined table salt. However, be aware that most commercial sea salt also contains anticaking agents. A better choice is unrefined sea salt made from evapo-rated seawater. Because our oceans are becoming more and more polluted, the source of this salt is important. See the list of resources at the back of the book for a reliable source.

• *Unrefined Rock Salt.* This type of salt is our choice. It has a cooling action, is diuretic, laxative, digestive, stimulating to the appetite and balancing for all three *doshas.* It is a pollutant free salt extracted in the United States from ancient seabeds and has a full complement of trace minerals. This salt is available in many natural food stores, or see the list of resources at the back of the book.

• *Bragg's Liquid Amino Acids.* Bragg's Liquid Amino Acids, a soy sauce alternative, contains a healthy source of sodium derived from soy protein. Most natural food stores carry this product.

• *Herbal Salts and Salt Free Herbal Seasonings.* Always read labels and choose a product that contains no MSG or other chemical addi-tives. Recommended herbal salts include Herbamare and Trocamare, made by Bioforce, available in natural food stores. Salt free herbal seasonings are also a good choice. There are many products available, or you can make your own by combining dried herbs to taste.

• *Salt Substitutes Made with Potassium Chloride.* These products contain the same undesirable chemical additives found in table salt and should be avoided. Potassium chloride is not utilized well by the body, and in large amounts may cause adverse reactions such as nausea, vomiting, diarrhea and ulcers.

• *Natural Foods.* We have said elsewhere in this book that we need to eat as close to nature as possible and this is certainly true with salt. Many foods contain natural sodium. Vegetables such as celery, carrots, beets, parsley, chard, kale and spinach all have a slightly salty flavor. The vegetable with the highest amount of natural sodium is celery. There is evidence that celery actually helps to lower high blood pressure, because it contains a compound called 3-n-butyl phthalide. Some holistic doctors suggest that hypertensive individuals eat four celery stalks per day.[32]

Foods that are processed or packaged contain much more sodium than those that are fresh and unprocessed. Stay away from chips, fries and frozen dinners. Natural foods also contain more of the essential nutrients our bodies require than foods that have been altered and processed. Remember that fresh is best, unprocessed frozen is next best, and processed or canned is least acceptable but perhaps better than nothing.

We do not need to consume salt that has added iodine in order to ensure proper functioning of the thyroid gland. Unrefined sea salt or rock salt, sometimes called mineral salt, contains trace amounts of naturally occurring iodine, as well as other essential trace minerals. Including these forms of salt along with iodine rich fish or sea vegetables, such as kelp, will more than meet your iodine needs.

One more suggestion: Put the salt you are using to the following test. Add a spoonful to a glass of plain water, stir it several times, and let it stand overnight. If the salt collects in a thick layer on the bottom of the glass, your salt has failed the test. This experiment gives a visual example of what refined salt can do to your system by collecting in the tissues and clogging the circulation. Unrefined natural salt will dissolve in a glass of water as well as in bodily fluids.[33] Your body can properly handle this type of unrefined salt.

Good Fats and Bad Fats

Good fats are anti-inflammatory and are good for the body. Bad fats create inflammation and lead to problems. Simply stated, good fats help the heart and bad fats damage it. Omega-3 fatty acids contained in fish oils, flaxseed oil and some nuts appear to protect against heart disease, especially sudden cardiac death. Omega-3s are called "essential fatty acids" because they can't be manufactured in the body and yet are essential elements in our diet. The American diet is alarmingly deficient in this important nutrient.

Fats are a confusing and often misunderstood aspect of our diet. There is an abundance of contradictory information about how much and what kind should be included in a health conscious diet, and it is difficult to know who is speaking the truth. The fact is that our bodies require a certain amount of fat to give us energy, help us absorb nutrients, provide thermal insulation, regulate our metabolism and maintain fertility. In addition, the heart uses fat as its main source of energy. But what kind of fat is best and how much is necessary?

Fat in our diet became the "Bad Guy" back in the 1970s when Nathan Pritikin, an avid medical researcher, began advocating an extremely low fat diet to treat heart disease. Pritikin's 1974 book, *Live Longer Now*, had a significant impact on dietary thinking in this country, and his message was echoed in the 1977 Dietary Goals for the United States.

The Pritikin prescription for optimal health was a low fat, low cholesterol, low sodium, high complex carbohydrate diet combined with regular aerobic exercise. He recommended only five to ten percent fat in the diet, and protein consumption was limited to a lean 3.5 ounces a day in order to reduce total fat and cholesterol intake.

In more recent years, Dr. Dean Ornish has advocated a similar approach to optimal health, including the same low percentage of fat. Both Pritikin and Ornish were able to achieve remarkable results in treating heart disease, and their approach has raised the awareness of the American public about the importance of proper food choices for health. We applaud the work of both these men.

However, the "truth" about fats has become muddled in recent years by research revealing that too little fat can be just as damaging as too much. Recently the American Heart Association warned that very low fat diets (less than 15 percent of total calories) tend to increase triglycerides and lower "good" cholesterol, possibly *raising* the risk of heart disease, and such a diet is not recommended for the population at large.[34]

Dr. Ornish, and Pritikin before him, never examined the difference between "good fats" and "bad fats." They lumped all fats together and labeled them as "bad." The secret to our search for the truth about this nutrient seems to lie in determining what fats are "good" and what fats are "bad." There is substantial evidence, which few would dispute, that diets high in saturated fat are unhealthy, because of their role in promoting inflammation and creating plaque that clogs the artieries. Our bodies cannot properly utilize saturated fats and, as a consequence, the fats tend to adhere to the walls of the blood vessels, leading to artheriosclorosis. However, we don't have comparable evidence that the percentage of *total* fat in the diet is equally determinative of health. In fact, there is emerging scientific consensus that the *kind* of fat we eat is at least as important as the amount.[35]

A recent article in *The New York Times Science Times*[36] reports that a growing number of nutrition, health and obesity specialists maintain that in trying to squeeze some of the heart damaging grease from our high fat diets, they have sent Americans the wrong message. "It's not fat per se that's the problem, the experts now say, but the kinds of fats Americans eat and the other kinds of foods they fill up on when they cut back on appetite satisfying fat." While heart disease has declined, obesity has risen by 50 percent since the big push to limit fat took off in the 1970s with the diets of Pritikin and Ornish. The ongoing Nurses Health Study has revealed that among 80,000 women total fat consumption did not affect coronary risk, but rather the kinds of fats the women ate.

A 1979 study investigated the diet of native Greenland Eskimos.[37] This study reported that despite an extremely high fat, high cholesterol diet, the Eskimos have a low incidence of coronary heart disease, diabetes and cancer. The key to the Eskimos' excellent health is the kind of fat they eat. Eskimos get their fat from marine life (seal, whale, walrus) and fatty cold water fish (herring, mackerel and salmon) that make up most of their diet. These foods contain oils which are high in two important Omega-3 fatty acids called eicosapentaenoic acid, or EPA, and docosahexenoic acid, or DHA. Omega-3 fatty acids in the form of EPA and DHA have been shown to protect the cardiovascular system.

As awareness was raised around the importance of including omega-3s in our diet, these oils became the wonder fats of the '90s. A recent study in the *Journal of the American Medical Association* suggests that eating fish at least once a week may *halve* the risk of sudden cardiac death. Other studies have shown omega-3s to lessen the clotting tendency of the blood, reduce heart arrhythmia and hypertension, improve rheumatoid arthritis, lower risk of kidney disease, and possibly protect against cancer. In addition, studies have indicated positive effects in combating psychiatric disorders, such as depression, bipolar disorder and even schizophrenia.[38] How have we overlooked this important nutrient for so long?

Another form of essential fatty acid, known as omega-6, is also important for health. However, this fat is much more available in our diet. We recommend that everyone supplement his/her diet each day with one to two tablespoons of cold pressed liquid flaxseed oil or its equivalent in gel caps, available in the refrigerated section of your natural food store. Flaxseed oil contains both omega-3s and omega-6s. Keep this oil cold. The oil can be taken either off the spoon or added to salads or other foods. Do not heat, because heat changes the nature of the oil.

What We Do to Fat. The real problem is not so much what fat does to us, but what we do to fat. The way we use or process fat is significant. Four factors to consider are heat, hydrogenation, oxidation and homogenization.

• *Heat.* Oils are commercially processed to improve shelf life, flavor, smell and color. Unfortunately, due to the high temperatures involved (sometimes up to 475 degrees), polyunsaturated fatty acids are converted from the naturally occurring, beneficial "cis" form to the unnatural, harmful "trans" form. Cis fats melt at 55 degrees, below the body temperature of 98.6, which makes them fully available to the system. Trans fats, on the other hand, melt at up to 111 degrees, so they remain solid and therefore unmetabolized in the human body.[39]

• *Hydrogenation.* The hydrogenation process converts liquid oils into hardened fats, such as margarine and vegetable shortening. This process destroys natural fatty acids by converting the natural form into the biologically impaired trans form, which strips the essential fatty acids of their biological potency. Trans fatty acids cannot be used properly by the body and furthermore impair the use of cis fatty acids.

Trans fatty acids and hydrogenated oils contribute to many disorders, including increased incidence of heart disease, increased levels of harmful cholesterol, increased cancer rates, increased prevalence of diabetes, increased incidence of obesity, immune suppression and essential fatty acid deficiencies. Many researchers and nutritionists have been concerned about the health effects of margarine since it first came on the market. Although many Americans assume they are eating more healthfully by consuming margarine instead of butter and saturated fats, in truth they may actually be doing more harm. Hydrogenated oils not only raise LDL cholesterol (the bad cholesterol), they also lower the protective HDL cholesterol level, interfere with essential fatty acid metabolism and are suspected of causing certain cancers.[40]

Trans fatty acids are rarely found in nature but are predominant in commercial salad oil (15 percent) and hydrogenated products such as margarine (30 percent) and shortening (47 percent).[41]

• *Oxidation.* Oxidation is a process during which toxins are formed by the combination of oxygen with other substances. The term antioxidant is used to denote a substance that protects against the process of oxidation. Antioxidant nutrients, such as beta-carotene, selenium, vitamin E and vitamin C, are important in protecting against the development of heart disease, cancer and other chronic degenerative diseases. In addition, antioxidants are thought to slow the aging process. Interaction with oxygen creates peroxides, or free radicals, that cause rancidity. The term "free radicals" has become synonymous with cell and tissue destruction. Premature aging, heart disease, cancer and other degenerative processes are the result of free radical activity.

Oils are more susceptible to oxygen once they have been extracted from their source. If you detect a rancid smell or taste, throw out the oil. The oxidation of oils is also related to temperature. Refrigerated oils do not become rancid as quickly as those left out at room temperature. Heated oils oxidize rapidly. At frying temperatures polyunsaturated oils not only rapidly oxidize but are also converted from the cis form to the trans form. The commercial practice of reusing frying oils raises the specter of both trans and oxidized fats to the most dangerous levels. The delicious french fries we love to eat are generally cooked in a chemical "soup" which is extremely toxic to the body. The oil is used over and over again at high heat, in addition to being filled with chemicals to extend the amount of time it can be used.

• *Homogenization.* Homogenization is another common technique that damages fats. Normal milk fat occurs in large globules that are usually digested intact in the intestinal tract. Homogenization breaks up these fat globules into extremely small droplets (one-third the original size) that are dispersed throughout the milk. These small droplets of fat are not readily digested.

Many homogenized fat particles bypass digestion and are absorbed directly into the bloodstream, carrying with them a destructive enzyme called xanthine oxidase (XO). As it is carried through the bloodstream, XO can damage the arteries and form lesions on artery walls, which then attract cholesterol and fat. Plaque buildup results.[42]

We recommend only nonfat milk and milk products. Without any fat, there is no XO that can be carried into the body's tissues. If you insist on using 2 percent or full-fat milk, boil it before drinking. Heat deactivates XO.[43]

Recognizing essential fatty acid deficiency. The signs and symptoms of essential fatty acid deficiency may be overt or chronically nagging and range from mild fatigue to fatal heart attack. Most Western physicians may never make an association between a health symptom and essential fatty acid deficiency; therefore, the underlying cause of illness continues to manifest. Most physicians are not trained in nutrition, and the laboratory analysis to measure essential fatty acid deficiency is not widely available or appreciated. In addition, the symptoms of essential fatty acid deficiency are not as obvious as those of some other nutrient deficiencies. The consequences, however, are far more deadly in this day and age. Even if an essential fatty acid deficiency were recognized, few orthodox clinicians would know how to treat it. The most damaging effects of essential fatty acid deficiency are inflammatory disease and plaque build up which precedes arteriosclerosis, high blood pressure (hypertension), heart attack and stroke.

In general, the symptoms of a deficiency of essential fatty acids can be so vague and broad that they are typically written off as something else. Suffice it to say, surveys suggest that Americans are up to 90 percent deficient in essential fatty acids. This simply means we are obtaining only 10 percent of what we need for optimal health.[44]

Some signs and symptoms of essential fatty acid deficiency include fatigue, malaise, lackluster energy; dry skin and hair; dry mucous membranes, tear ducts, mouth and vagina; improper digestion, gas, bloating; constipation; immune weakness; depression; high blood pressure; arthritis.

Choosing Your Oils. Although there is still debate about what kinds of oils are safe to use, some choices are widely accepted:
• ***Ghee.*** We recommend *ghee*. We think it is the only fat that does not break down with high heat. Use *ghee* for sautés and stirfrys. Although butter, from which *ghee* is made, burns with high heat, butter has health benefits. Among other things, it contains butyric

acid, a short chain fatty acid, which supports the friendly bacteria of the colon.

• *Olive Oil*. Cold pressed extra virgin olive oil is excellent for salads and low heat cooking but will break down with high heat.

• *Flaxseed oil*. We have already talked about the health benefits of flaxseed oil and the importance of including one to two tablespoons each day in your diet. This oil should not be heated, beacuse it breaks down easily with heat.

If you choose to use sunflower oil, safflower oil or peanut oil, be cautious of your source. Be sure these oils have not been refined or heated before bottling. They will break down and form free radicals with high heat. Canola oil is often recommended for cooking. However, we feel canola is an inferior oil. Like soybean oil, it is sometimes partially hydrogenated to prevent "off flavors" from forming. In addition, rapeseed, from which it is made, is widely grown with heavy applications of pesticides. If you choose to use canola, select one that is organic and not hydrogenated.

Avoid:
• Margarine
• Any hydrogenated oil
• Saturated animal fats, such as lard
• Any rancid fats

* * * * *

We do have a choice in the foods we eat, and this is one area over which we have control. Food nourishes our total being and is our best medicine, both for prevention and for treatment. If food choices are not made with awareness, treatment with herbs and supplements will do little for us.

Our food choices are vital for maintaining balance. Raising awareness around the way different foods affect us in maintaining balance as we "ride" the bike of life is the first step to vital health, longevity and quality of life in body, mind and consciousness.

CHAPTER 11

Managing Your Environment
So It Doesn't Make You Toxic

We have control over what we eat. However, when it comes to the environment, we are faced with more difficult situations, some over which we have little control.

In this chapter we will consider:
- **The importance of water**
- **Exercise and its impact on immunity**
- **Stress and the development of disease**
- **Light and sleep**
- **Airborne pollution**
- **Background radiation**

Water

How Much Water? How much water should you drink each day? Many, including Dr. Lad, suggest seven to eight glasses on average each day. In a hot humid climate when sweating, more is needed. More is also needed in a hot dry climate. Too much water, more than your body can process, can decrease kidney energy due to excess strain on the kidneys to deal with the liquid. Some people drink a gallon or more a day, thinking that the water will cleanse their systems. However, this is far too much for most people and may cause more harm than good. If you suffer from edema or facial puffiness, cut back on water intake and see if the condition corrects itself. Stay alert to your body's needs. More is not necessarily better.

Imagine for a moment a clear mountain stream. You can see right to the bottom. Beavers come and drop a log to dam the stream. Behind the dam water starts to back up. Silt falls to the bottom, algae grows, and pretty soon a scum forms on top of the pond and mosquitoes begin to breed. What had been a clear stream is now a sludgy pond with mosquitoes.

If you think about your body as that stream, without enough water you will create an environment that will lead to disease. Like the beaver pond, your liquid flow can become stagnant. You need to flush through every day. You need to keep your cells clean rather than let your tissues get clogged up, which creates ill health.[1]

Disease may be caused by a buildup of toxins in the tissues. If the "flowing water" of your body is not kept running smoothly, you will develop sludge (toxins) just as surely as the beaver pond. Drinking an adequate amount of water each day is important and contributes to health.

What Type of Water? What type of water should you drink? Your body needs pure water of the highest quality. There are many forms of filtration. Perhaps the best is reverse osmosis (RO) available from the many clean water stores now open across the country. There are also many home filters on the market, ranging in price from several hundred dollars down. If all you can afford is something like a Brita or some other brand of small water filter, choose that.

Carbonation. Artificially carbonated water, water that has bubbles added, uses benzene, a known carcinogen, to create the bubbles. We do not know what the long term effects are of low level doses of carcinogens. Perhaps no one source is a cancer culprit, but when our water, our drinks, and our food all regularly contain low levels of carcinogens for bubbles or flavor, we choose to recommend caution. The newspapers noted recently a product recall by a number of soft drink and bottled water companies. Because of an error in the equipment that added carbonation, more benzene entered the water than usual. The product recall said, "There has been an unsafe level of the carcinogen benzene released into Coca-Cola, 7-Up and several other soft drinks and bottled waters." Millions of bottles and cans were recalled. An unsafe level of the carcinogen benzene? How much is safe? It is just one more chemical for your body's immune system to deal with.[2]

Fluoridation. Fluoride decreases white blood cell activity as much as sugar does. The story on fluoride is controversial. The studies showing that fluoride might be beneficial in managing dental disease were carried out on water that had *calcium fluoride* in it. However, it is *sodium fluoride* that is added to water supplies—one more source of sodium! The safe limit for added flouride is considered to be 1 to 4 ppm. However, flouride is routinely added up to 1100 ppm, presumably because it leaches out in transit through the pipes. We then get additional fluoride in our toothpaste or mouthwash, which travels through the mucous membrane of the mouth into the bloodstream. There is strong evidence that the modern improvement in dental health may have little to do with fluoride added to our water. There are communities where fluoride has never been added where dental health has improved at the same rate as in communities where it has been added. Our improved dental health probably has more to do with better choices of food, exercise and lifestyle than with flouride.[3]

Tap Water. What about tap water? It depends on where you are and the source of the water. Margaret's tap water comes from a 420-foot well in rural Maine. This water, which has been tested, is pure and safe. However, recently several cities in this country have reported polluted water, which included heavy metals such as arsenic and mercury. We need good water and plenty of it to support the immune system. The amount and type of water we drink is one more area over which we have control.

What happens if you don't get enough water? We have always known that we need water to survive. However, recent research seems to indicate that chronic dehydration may be a root cause of many of our disease conditions. We need sufficient water to flush toxins from our cells.[4]

Tea, coffee, alcohol and manufactured beverages are not desirable substitutes for the natural water needs of our bodies. It is true that these beverages contain water, but other ingredients in these drinks can cause dehydration. They remove the water in which they are dissolved, plus additional water from the reserves of the body. Children today are not educated to drink water and become dependent on sodas and juices. A cultivated preference for the taste of these other liquids reduces the urge to drink water even when sodas and juices are not available.[5]

Awareness of dehydration is particularly important during periods of high heat, especially in the desert. As the summer heat began to descend on the Phoenix area, where we wrote the first draft of this book, *The Arizona Republic* ran a lengthy front page article on the dangers of dehydration.[6] "The odds are you're dehydrated and don't know it. Valley health professionals estimate that two of three Arizonans drink far too little water." Where there is triple-digit heat, people need to be particularly aware of dehydration. Signals of dehydration include heartburn, stomach pain, non-infectious recurring or chronic pain, low back pain, headache, mental irritation, depression, and fatigue. Included under "Advanced Dehydration/Heatstroke" are nausea, diarrhea, severe muscle cramping, dizziness, fainting, disorientation, and even seizures.[7]

Extreme, we might say? Or is it? Look carefully at the results of dehydration. Dehydration and disease go together. Without sufficient water in our systems to flush out toxins, they remain in our cells and create disease. A study published in the *New England Journal of Medicine* found that drinking more fluids, particularly water, could lower the risk of bladder cancer. "Some researchers believe the bladder lining suffers less exposure to cancer causing substances in urine when the urine is diluted and urination is more frequent."[8]

Because of a gradually failing thirst sensation, our bodies become chronically and increasingly dehydrated as we age. With increase in age, the water content of the cells of the body decreases, to the point where the ratio of the volume of water that is inside the cells to that outside the cells may change drastically. As a result, chronic dehydration can lead to disease when the emergency signals of dehydration are not understood.[9] Humans seem to lose their thirst sensation and the critical perception of needing water. Not recognizing their water need, they become gradually, increasingly and chronically dehydrated with age.[10]

A recent article by Jane Brody reported that "older people have a reduced thirst mechanism—they have to consciously think of drinking more and keeping well hydrated, especially if they live in warm climates." The new food-guide pyramid revised for seniors over 70 recommends eight glasses of water each day (64 ounces).[11]

A dry mouth is an advanced sign of dehydration. The body can suffer from dehydration even when the mouth is fairly moist. Still worse, in the elderly, the mouth may be obviously dry and yet thirst may not be acknowledged and satisfied.[12] The thirst sensation is lost, because the body's intelligence is covered over by imbalanced *doshas* and accumulation of toxins, both of which could be helped by the consumption of water.

The need for water is critical for a strong immune response. Drink the best quality water you can access in the amount appropriate for you.

Glass versus Plastic. There are certain types of plastic bottles used by water companies that are designed not to leach. However, plastics are made from volatile compounds. Not all plastic water bottles are safe.

According to a growing body of evidence, the chemicals that make up many plastics may migrate out of them and into foods and fluids, ending up in our bodies. In a recent issue of *Time* the dangers of plastics were discussed.[13] The medical community is beginning to listen. The plastic products most suspect are those made of a material known as polyvinyl chloride, or PVC. This plastic is made pliable by the addition of softeners that easily leach out. Animal studies indicate that these softeners can damage the liver, heart, kidneys and testicles and may cause cancer. Millions of IV bags made of PVC are used each year in this country. The article in *Time* also raised the question of the safety of plastic wraps used in food storage. Plastic toys, which spend so much time in the mouths of babies, are also a concern, as are plastic baby bottles and nipples.[14]

We are "addicted" to the convenience of plastics. Perhaps we are not willing to give up this convenience. However, at least raise awareness around the possible dangers involved and substitute glass or ceramic whenever possible. Margaret likes good old waxed paper, which works fine for many things.

The water companies don't have much choice. If they used ceramic or glass, it would be impractical. If you buy filtered water in plastic or have it delivered, try to keep the time in the plastic as short as possible. If you plan to store drinking water for any length of time, use glass or ceramic.

Lifestyle

Exercise. Exercise is another important way to enhance your immune function. It increases the body's capacity to perform physical tasks, promotes mental and emotional clarity and improves digestion. Exercise produces a feeling of lightness in the body. By stimulating circulation, it helps to transform toxins into less harmful substances and aids in removing them from the system. The delivery of white blood cells around the body is enhanced when you exercise and move the blood. Blood stasis is often the cause of disease, and we can change stagnation by exercising. We evolved to run or walk between 10 to 20 miles a day while hunting and gathering. The chair was only created about 3000 years ago. Before the chair, we squatted or sat on the ground. Even after the chair was created, we were quite physically active. Only in the last hundred years or so since the car came along have we physically slowed down. Our lifestyles have become sedentary at home and at work.

Getting on a good exercise program as part of your healing path can make a difference in the way you feel. Exercising outdoors is ideal. In an environment of fresh air, you will deliver more oxygen to your body. Viruses, bacteria, microbes do not like oxygen and operate inefficiently in a high oxygen environment. If you can't exercise, at least open the window and take some good deep breaths. Most of us only use about 15 to 20 percent of our lung capacity. We should breathe much more deeply, belly breathing, down to the base of our lungs, and that alone would help the immune system. It sounds simple, but it really works.

In addition, while exercising outdoors, you expose youself to the sun. The sun has had bad press over the last several years. However, there are important things that the sun does for you, specifically for your immune system. Again, viruses, bacteria, fungi, various microbes are damaged by ultraviolet light. In fact, ultraviolet is used as a disinfectant. Sunlight supports the immune function. SAD (seasonal affective disorder), a type of depression, is widespread in areas where sunshine is limited. We feel better when the sun is out. The sun livens and brightens us.[15] So use a little sunscreen and get outdoors.

Choose an exercise program that works for you. Walking is excellent and almost everyone can get out and move. Swimming is also highly recommended. Margaret broke her leg several years ago, and water aerobics worked wonders in regaining the use of the leg. Water exercise is also quite helpful for people with such conditions as multiple sclerosis or arthritis, who may find walking difficult. Although swimming is acceptable for all three constitutions—*vata, pitta* and *kapha*—it is especially recommended for a *vata* or for someone with a *vata* imbalance. *Vata* is dry and light and water is wet and heavy. We do not recommend jogging, especially for *vata* dominant individuals, because of its impact on the joints.

For those for whom strenuous exercise is not possible or desirable, we recommend T'ai Chi Chuan. This ancient Chinese exercise is performed in slow, relaxed, continuous movements, which energize the body. A recent newspaper article reported that T'ai Chi "is just as effective in reducing blood pressure as aerobic workouts." The article cited a study which followed 62 sedentary adults age 60 and older who wanted to lower their blood pressure. T'ai Chi can also improve balance and is easy on the joints.[16]

Yoga is another discipline we highly recommend. Yoga classes are now widely available. Shop around until you find a teacher who appeals to you. We underestimate the importance of stretching. It's the part of our exercise routine that most of us are tempted to skip. Yet, the more exercise physiologists learn about stretching—which causes the ligaments, tendons and muscles to lengthen—the more benefits they find. Stretching reduces stress and feelings of fatigue and increases strength. It increases awareness and skill in action. It helps maintain flexibility and range of motion, eases muscle soreness and improves recovery time. Flexibility of body means flexibility of mind. Yoga is much more than physical exercise and stretching. It addresses the whole person—body, mind and consciousness. With expanded consciousness, we have a greater capacity for transcendental experiences.

Whatever you decide to do, stick with it. Exercise is another health factor over which we have control.

Stress. The damaging effects of stress cannot be overemphasized. Stress erodes the immune system and sets us up for disease. Examine the stresses in your life. Although stress is real, many times we can modify how we respond in a situation by becoming aware of the relationship between outside pressures and our inner dialogue, and by learning stress reducing techniques, including exercise. Have you ever noticed how people respond differently to the same situation? If you can't modify your own inner response to alleviate stress, deal with it in some other way. If it is a troubling relationship or work situation, get out of it. If you can't remove yourself from a situation, increased awareness and relaxation techniques can be helpful.

If you live in fear of being overwhelmed or pressured, of being unable to perform adequately, your emotions and nervous system will feel agitated. If the emotions do not get resolved, the nervous system will send messages to your body for help and it will respond. What part of the body responds will be determined in part by the nature of the stress. For example, those with an overdeveloped sense of responsibility hold tension in their shoulders, which become hard and stiff. When heavy responsibility comes to an end, we often say "I feel as if I have just had a thousand pounds lifted from my shoulders." Those who feel threatened or defeated by life often have lower back pains and are advised by their friends to "stand up and show a little backbone." Different types of stress act on different areas of the body. Unresolved emotional issues become "calcified" in the body and become a major source of energetic and physical imbalance. Even Western science has come to recognize this phenomenon.[17]

What is to be done to change your reaction to stress? Quieting the mind so that it is not in a state of constant agitation provides one of the most important keys. When operating from calmness, notice that your energy does not feel drained, your emotions remain calm and you do not accumulate stress in your mind or body even though there may be many demands on you.

Only when you feel calm and focused are you able to exercise control over your reactions to pressing external demands without feeling stressed. To achieve that state takes us to matters of "spirit," to how we relate to our universe. Much of our need to control events and to control others is based on feelings of super-responsibility, distrust, fear, non-support, etc.

Some people learn to calm their minds through different forms of meditation or relaxation exercises. Others use yoga or other forms of exercise. Still others rely on spiritual beliefs and devotional practices. One need only think of Mahatma Ghandi, Mother Teresa, the Dalai Lama or Dr. Martin Luther King as examples of people who managed to maintain extraordinary levels of calmness is spite of extreme external pressures. Each of them used devotional practices to achieve calmness. They all sought to improve their worlds through a combination of devotional practices and practical actions. Each learned to transcend fear and exhibited inner qualities of strength, devotion and peace of mind amid incredible poverty, oppression, discrimination, and economic and political turmoil. In each there was an integration of body, mind and consciousness. Regardless of your personal religious or spiritual beliefs, there are paths to calming the mind that can be helpful to you. Which path you select depends on your own preferences.

Stress is an idea within your mind that creates biological and chemical reactions in your body. When you cannot control the external events, you can learn to calm your mind and control your internal reactions.

Environment

Light and Sleep. Both light and sleep are critical for immune health. We have discussed the healing values of sunlight. Now let's look at the effects of different kinds of artificial lighting on our health.

Artificial lighting, especially fluorescent lighting, is harmful. There is a flicker in fluorescent lighting that is quite tiring to the eyes and can cause headaches. Being under any kind of artificial lighting disrupts our pineal gland function. The pineal gland is sometimes called the vestigial third eye. It is deep inside and maintains a relationship with light through the eyes. The pineal gland affects all the rhythmic processes in the body, which ultimately include the pituitary gland function. The pineal gland affects the sleep/wake cycle and the cyclical processes of every organ in the body.

When we are exposed to artificial light, the pineal function is disrupted. Melatonin is produced by the pineal gland in the dark, in the absence of light. Years ago we used to go to bed at sundown and get up at sunrise. There were candles and oil lamps but the light was of poor quality. On the average, 200 years ago we slept two hours longer each night. It is important that we get that sleep, especially the sleep that happens in the early morning between 3:00 AM and 5:00 AM. There is a surge of melatonin at that time. Under the influence of that hormone, we release another hormone from the pituitary called growth hormone. In children and young people, growth hormone promotes growth of the body. In adults it actually switches on the immune function for the immune system to heal itself.

If we either don't sleep soundly, or if we sleep in a room that is not completely dark, we inhibit the release of melatonin. There should be no streetlights shining in, no night light on the wall and no electric clock that shines all night. Sleep in the darkest room possible.[18]

Airborne Pollution. Airborne pollution is also a factor that impacts negatively on the immune system. There is quite a bit you can do about this pollution in your own home. Common home pollutants that carry airborne particles to which many are allergic include formaldehyde and lacquer. Ideally, use natural fabrics and natural building materials that do not emit toxic fumes. If that isn't possible, air filters and vacuum sweepers can help remove fumes, dust mites and allergens. Cleaning the ducts in your house can also help.

We have less control over pollution outside our homes or in the workplace. We can work for legislation to clean up the environment or try to choose a work environment that is healthy. However, our control in these situations may be limited.

Concern regarding airborne pollution is growing and awareness about its danger to our health is gradually taking hold. Much can be found in the press regarding these issues. For example, a recent article reported that air pollution in Southern California appears to have subtle, long-term effects on children's lungs.[19] TV stations now commonly give smog alerts, urging people, especially children, to stay indoors to avoid respiratory problems. We can only hope that public awareness will continue to rise and that much needed action will be taken to clean up this dangerous threat to our immunity.

Background Radiation. Some background radiation is natural and inevitable. The earth gives off radon gas. There are pockets where it is more concentrated, but we are exposed to it all the time. However, there are other sources of background radiation and ionizing radiation that are quite damaging to the immune system. Things like fluorescent lights, television screens, computer monitors, digital clocks and microwave ovens all give off electromagnetic frequencies and background radiation. You have a choice and you could just not use those things. You could go back to the last century and live that way, but most of us are not willing to give up our conveniences, so we need to do things to protect ourselves.

There are things you can do. If you use a digital electric clock in your bedroom, don't sleep with it next to your head. Move it across the room.

The same is true with cordless telephones. The batteries in these phones give off radiation and, although they are handy gadgets, having them close to us as we sleep is not a good idea. Cell phones are even more damaging. We do not like microwaves and refuse to be in a kitchen if one is in use. Frankly, we feel it saps our energy. Choosing not to use a microwave is not a hardship. There are alternatives.

We live in a polluted world. There are some factors over which we have control and some we don't. When it comes to diet, water, exercise and many other lifestyle decisions, we need to choose for health. If we support our immune system and work to maintain our state of balance in ways over which we have control, we will be better able to withstand the assault of those factors over which we have no control.

CHAPTER 12

THE EXTRA TOUCH FOR IMMUNITY: ENHANCING BALANCE WITH HERBS AND SUPPLEMENTS

THERE IS MORE THAT WE CAN DO to help maintain a smooth "ride" of balance on the bike of life. In addition to choices of food, lifestyle and exercise, many common herbs, spices and easily available supplements can make the "ride" easier.

In this chapter we will discuss herbs to support immunity and maintain balance, including:
  * **Kitchen medicine**
  * **Surface and deep immune stimulants**
  * **Supplements for a strong immunity**

Kitchen Medicine

Many common herbs found in most kitchens are more powerful substances than we have realized. Their power to maintain health and restore balance is being rediscovered. The knowledge and usage of everything in this section goes back thousands of years, and the safety and effectiveness of these herbs have been proven by time.

Garlic. Garlic, that stinky little clove, has been valued for its medicinal qualities for thousands of years and is recently being rediscovered and proven through modern scientific studies. The medicinal qualities of garlic have yet to be identified, and modern scientists keep changing their minds about exactly what is the active ingredient. The bottom line is, the whole plant is always better than any isolated constituent.

Garlic is antiviral, antibacterial and antifungal. Scientific studies have pointed to its help in reducing cholesterol and normalizing blood pressure. Its essential properties seem to be carried in the volatile oil, and cooking your garlic is not the best thing to do when taking it as a medicine. It is much better to take it raw. When you add garlic to the pan and cook it, the entire kitchen fills with its distinctive smell. That smell is a result of the release of the volatile oils, through which many of the medicinal properties are lost. By all means use garlic in cooking—in stirfrys, soups, sauces and stews—and use plenty of it. But let's also talk about how to use it raw.

Won't we drive everyone away if we eat raw garlic? Try taking it this way: Peel a clove of garlic and chop it up. Put it on a spoon and place it on the back of your tongue, as if you were swallowing a pill. Wash it down with water without chewing. If you take it in this way at night, by morning the offensive smell will have dispersed. If you sleep with a partner, it might be well to enlist that person's cooperation and even participation.

Garlic in vinegar also works and this combination can be added to salads or vegetables. Garlic honey is delicious. Chop up some garlic cloves. Put them in a jar and cover with raw honey. Let the mixture sit for a couple of weeks and then strain. This combination can also be used in salad dressing. However, remember, never use honey in cooking or baking.

A number of odorless garlic capsules are available. There is debate about the effectiveness of these products, and they are expensive. It is certainly better to take these capsules than not to consume garlic at all. However, being aware of the health benefits of fresh garlic, we need to find a way to incorporate this valuable substance into our diet.[1]

Garlic has a pungent taste, is heating, with a pungent post-digestive effect. It qualities are oily and heavy. It calms *vata* and *kapha* and increases *pitta*. The term "post-digestive effect" refers to the taste and action of a substance after the completion of the digestive process

Onions (*Allium cepa*). The common onion is packed with medicinal qualities for better health. All members of the onion family share certain key qualities: they are pungent and influence the lungs; they promote warmth and thus move energy in the body, resolve stagnation, reduce clotting, and expel coldness. They are perhaps the foods richest in sulfur, a warming element that purifies the body, helps remove heavy metals and parasites, and facilitates protein/amino acid metabolism. Onions clean the arteries and retard the growth of viruses, yeasts and other pathogenic organisms.[2]

Onions lower blood pressure and cholesterol and decrease phlegm and inflammation of the nose and throat. They inhibit allergic reactions, induce sweating, and help in treating the common cold. Yellow onions contain quercitin, a substance believed to inhibit allergies.

Cooked onions have a sweet taste, are slightly heating, and have a sweet post-digestive effect. The actions are digestive and carminative. Cooked onions are calming to all *doshas*. Their actions of raw onions are heavy and appetizing. Raw onions increase *vata* and *pitta* because of their pungent taste and decrease *kapha* because they are heating.

Turmeric (*Curcuma longa*). Turmeric has a long tradition of usage in Ayurvedic medicine. Turmeric helps digestion, maintains the flora of the intestine, reduces gas and has tonic properties. It acts as an antibiotic, antifungal and is an effective anti-cancer agent. Its action is also anti-inflammatory. Its bright yellow color stains, so be careful not to get it on your clothes. Hydrogen peroxide in wash water helps remove stains.

Turmeric, along with cumin, coriander and mustard seeds, can easily be added to stirfry dishes.[3] It does have a strong taste, so start with a small amount and build slowly.

For a delicious bedtime drink, bring one cup of milk and one-half teaspoon of turmeric to a boil. Pour into a cup and sip. The medicinal qualities of the turmeric and the calming effects of the milk will bring deep sleep. Like coffee, the taste is acquired, but once acquired is truly enjoyed.

Turmeric is bitter, heating, with a pungent post-digestive effect, and is balancing for all three *doshas*. Excessive use may increase *pitta*. Its actions are dry, light and digestive.

Vinegar. In the early years of the twentieth century, Dr. D. C. Jarvis of Barre, Vermont, wrote a little book called *Vermont Folk Medicine*, in which he outlined the health benefits of apple cider vinegar. Dr. Jarvis noted how potassium in its natural combination with other trace minerals is essential to the metabolic process in every form of life on earth, and how without it there would be no life. One of the functions of potassium in our systems is to keep the tissues soft and pliable. Potassium is to the soft tissues what calcium is to the bone tissues. Hardening of the arteries takes place more readily in the presence of a deficiency of potassium. Apple cider vinegar is an excellent source of potassium and many minerals necessary for tissue health. It is also helpful in maintaining a balanced metabolism.

Apple cider vinegar has been found to affect the body's acid/alkaline balance as an alkaline food. The organic acids of the vinegar are oxidized in the body to furnish energy and leave an alkaline base residue in the blood, leading to the formation of urine that is less acid. Apples safeguard the body against acidosis and its ailments, such as indigestion, gout, ulcers, gas and bloating, and their properties carry over into the vinegar. The malic acid content of apples dissolves calcium deposits, and the alkaline residue left by this acid-rich vinegar aids in recovery from colds, flu, virus infections and hangovers. The acid in apple cider vinegar has also been credited with cures for arthritis, rheumatism and kidney stones, because of its ability to dissolve calcium crystals.

What exactly does apple cider vinegar do? In folk medicine its values are lauded.

> It favors oxidation of the blood; it tends to prevent intestinal putrefaction; it regulates calcium metabolism; it retards the onset of old age; it renders the urine normal, thus counteracting the too frequent urge to urinate; it affects the blood, making it of the right consistency; it regulates menstruation, and hence is very beneficial for women; it cures and prevents obesity; it promotes digestion, for the reason that cider vinegar bears a closer resemblance to the digestive juices than does any other liquid. And so, taking all in all, though it may not be a universal panacea, it is a polychrest of such extensive range if taken in the manner hereafter to be indicated, that, fearing to overtax credulity, I would hesitate to place the facts before the public, were it not . . . that people who take an intelligent interest in matters of health are more and more coming to the conclusion that disease is a unity, and hence that a number of apparently disconnected diseases have but one prime cause.[4]

Because of its effect on metabolism, this old Vermont folk remedy has been found helpful in controlling obesity. Dr. Jarvis suggests taking two teaspoons of cider vinegar and one teaspoon of honey in a glass of water each morning on an empty stomach. According to Ayurveda, honey also has an effect on controlling excess weight, because of its scraping action.

Be sure to choose organic, raw and unfiltered apple cider vinegar, because other forms of vinegar—white vinegar, wine vinegar, etc.—do not have the same medicinal effect. Read the label carefully. Once a bottle has been opened, keep it in the refrigerator and shake before using.

Vinegar decreases *vata* and *kapha* and increases *pitta*.

Honey. Honey in small amounts is a good form of sweetener, especially for a *kapha* individual. In the section above, we talked about the scraping action of honey and how it may be beneficial for weight reduction. A recommended drink, especially for *kapha*, is a cup of hot water with lemon and honey. A word of warning: Honey should not be cooked. Be sure your water is not too hot when you add the honey, because heat can cause honey to break down.

Never cook with honey. Heat changes honey to a substance the body can't deal with, and therefore stores as toxic buildup. Read the labels on breads and cereals you buy. Many of these products contain cooked honey that should be avoided.

Choose honey that is raw and unfiltered, because processing changes its properties. Those who suffer from allergies may find it beneficial to choose a local honey, made by bees from plants of the area. Taking this honey may help to desensitize to these plants.

Honey has a sweet taste, is heating, with a sweet post-digestive effect. Its actions are strengthening and heavy. It calms *vata* and increases *pitta*. In moderation it decreases *kapha,* and in excess it increases *kapha*.

Ginger (*Zingibar officinale*). An herbal medicine chest without ginger would be incomplete. It is perhaps the best of the spices and has been called the universal medicine. Ginger can be used for arthritic conditions and is a tonic for the heart. It relieves gas and cramps in the abdomen, including menstrual cramps due to cold. Externally, it makes a good paste for pain and headache.[5]

Dried ginger powder is hotter than the fresh ginger rhizome. It is a better stimulant and expectorant for reducing *kapha* and increasing digestive fire. The powder should be used with care, if at all, by those with high *pitta*. The fresh root can be used by all three *doshas*.

Fresh ginger is pungent, heating, with a sweet post-digestive effect. Its actions are light, juicy and digestive. It calms *vata* and *kapha* and decreases *pitta* initially. Excessive usage may increase *pitta*.

Green Tea (*Camellia thea sinesis*). Green tea has become a popular choice in the West only within the last few years. Recent scientific research has revealed that tea, and especially green tea, has an anti-cancer action that is quite significant. Green tea is widely available in supermarkets. If you have access to an oriental market, we recommend Gunpowder Tea, packaged in a green box.

Hawthorn (*Crataegus oxycanthus*). Many varieties of Hawthorn grow in our yards both in this country and in Europe. These plants range in size from a small bush to a large tree. All varieties of hawthorn have medicinal properties, some more than others. In Europe Hawthorn berries have been used as a food for thousands of years.

Hawthorn is a food for the heart and is helpful for any cardiac condition. It is quite safe and can be taken as a preventive for heart disease. Hawthorn helps prevent the oxidative process in the body and increases peripheral circulation. It is anti-inflammatory, anti-allergic, antiviral and anti-carcinogenic. By increasing blood supply to the coronary vessels, improving heart muscle contraction, and eliminating rhythm disturbances, Hawthorn is effective in reducing blood pressure, angina attacks and deposits of cholesterol. It is also an antispasmodic sedative.

Although the Hawthorn berry is widely used, the leaf and flower of the plant are also active medicinally.

If you have a Hawthorn in your yard, you can make your own jam from the berries. Otherwise, examine the many Hawthorn products in your natural food store. Many herbalists feel that the average American should take Hawthorn on a daily basis as a tonic.

If you are taking a digitalis based drug or a beta blocker, Hawthorn may potentiate the effect of the drug. Work with your doctor to modify and lower the dose of these drugs. Otherwise, Hawthorn is extremely safe with no side effects.[6]

Hawthorn is sour and heating with a sour post-digestive effect. It decreases *vata* and increases *pitta*. In excess it also increases *kapha*.

Herbs for Immunity

The usage of herbs has become increasingly popular over recent years. We look on the shelves of our natural food stores and are overwhelmed by the choices available. We don't know what to buy and we certainly don't know how safe the herbs are. A number of recent articles in *The New York Times* have cautioned about using herbs, because of unknown effects.[7] Even *Time*, the popular news magazine, ran a cover story on "The Herbal Medicine Boom," in which it cautioned about using substances about which we know so little.[8]

Herbs are powerful substances and are not to be taken lightly. Margaret will always remember her first class in Chinese Herbal Medicine, taught by Ted Kaptchuk, a Doctor of Oriental Medicine, in which Ted said that we need to know what we are doing when we treat with herbs. If we don't have the knowledge to properly use herbal substances, we can make people worse.

All of the herbs suggested in this book are safe for most people. As with food, water or anything we put into our bodies, we need to be aware of how our individual bodies are reacting. Some of us are much more sensitive than others. Respect what your body says to you.

With these words of caution, let's look at some of the herbs available to help us keep our immunity functioning well.

Surface Immune Stimulants for Acute Conditions.

Surface immune stimulants are used for conditions that come on quickly, what we call acute conditions. Such disorders would include a cold or flu. The herbs most effective for such conditions stimulate the white blood cells to attack invaders and restore balance. These herbs should be taken short term, only until the acute condition disappears.

Echinacea (*E. angustifolia* or *E. purpurea*). Echinacea is a Native American herb that has been used for thousands of years. It increases white blood cell activity and is anti-bacterial and anti-viral. When used as a single herb, it is most effective as a preventative taken at the beginning of an illness. Echinacea is called for when you have an achy feeling at night with the thought that you're going to wake up sick in the morning. If this herb is taken at the beginning, it can usually prevent development of achy or stuffy feelings. Take a teaspoon of the tincture and go to bed. If you still don't feel well the next morning, continue taking the tincture three or four times throughout the day. Take this herb only until acute symptoms disappear.

Tieraona Low Dog, a medical doctor and herbalist in Albuquerque, New Mexico, says that Echinacea is safe in large doses. As a Lakota Indian, she grew up with this herb. For acute conditions, she recommends taking a teaspoon of the tincture each hour until symptoms lessen. Then reduce the amount and continue until symptoms disappear. Again, listen to your body for the amount appropriate for you.

Echinacea is safe for children in a reduced amount relative to the age of the child. Tinctures made with vegetable glycerin are available for children. These tinctures taste good and avoid the alcohol contained in other tinctures. Although glycerin does not extract the medicinal qualities of an herb as well as alcohol, it is still a good choice, especially for children.

Although Echinacea root is most often used medicinally, the flowers and leaves are also useful. A product available from HerbPharm called Super Echinacea contains the root, flowers and leaves and works quite effectively. This product is available in most natural food stores. Echinacea also works synergistically with other antibiotic herbs, such as Goldenseal or Garlic.

Echinacea is bitter and pungent, is cooling and has a pungent post-digestive effect. It increases *vata* and decreases *pitta* and *kapha*.

Goldenseal (*Hydrastis canadensis*). In recent years Goldenseal has become almost as popular as Echinacea. Its actions are anti-bacterial, anti-viral, anti-fungal and anti-inflammatory. Goldenseal is cooling, making it helpful in illnesses with fever and hot irritations. Energetically, goldenseal is a cool, damp herb and it combines well with dry and hot herbs, such as Cayenne and Ginger.

Goldenseal is a threatened species and is not yet widely cultivated. Most of the Goldenseal available in the marketplace is wildcrafted and there is very little of it left. Therefore, use this herb consciously and only when some other herb will not work for you.

Goldenseal is powerful and is not for long term use. It can safely be used for 14 days on, then 14 days off.

Goldenseal is bitter and astringent, cooling, with a pungent post-digestive effect. It is perhaps the strongest anti-*pitta* herb available in this country.[9]

Usnea (*Usnea barbata*). In contrast to Goldenseal, Usnea is widely available in nature. It is a lichen that grows throughout northern Europe and across Russia. This herb contains usnic acid, a strong stimulator of white blood cell activity, and has some specific anti-bacterial activity. Although it is a lesser known herb in this country, it was recommended by early Chinese and Greek herbalists and was used in the Civil War to pack wounds to prevent infection. There are many products in Europe that contain Usnea. It is effective topically for impetigo, ringworm and athletes foot. Usnea affects the urinary, respiratory and digestive tracts and is indicated for any bacterial infection in those systems, including sinus infections, bronchitis, urethritis and cystitis.

Osha (*Ligusticum porteri*). Osha contains volatile oils and is a warming herb that helps to loosen mucus that is stuck and stagnant in the lower part of the lungs. It helps to bring this mucus up and out. Osha has some antibiotic and antibacterial activity, but is most effective for chronic lung infections that have gone deep, where a person is coughing but not productive. When material is coughed up, it is thick, sticky, and hard to move.

Osha is pungent and bitter, heating, with a pungent post-digestive effect. It decreases *kapha* and *vata* and increases *pitta*.

Garlic. And don't forget Garlic, which we have already discussed.

Deep Immune Support for Long Term Use

In contrast to the surface immune stimulants for acute conditions, herbs for deep immune support work in a different way. These herbs work slowly at the cellular level to increase the vitality in our life force energy, our immune function and the strength of our adrenals. We have already discussed how Echinacea activates white blood cells already present in the system. In contrast, the herbs in this section don't change the way the white blood cells function but simply provide more of them. Taking one of these herbs when you feel you are "coming down with something" won't keep you from getting sick. That's when you need Echinacea. However, if you are a person who frequently gets colds or flu, or if you have an immune dysfunction or allergies, the herbs in this section are the ones to choose to strengthen your immunity. They work over the long term and gently at a deep level.

Ginseng. Everyone has heard of Ginseng, and we look on it as the ultimate tonic herb. Korean Ginseng (*Panax ginseng*) is quite strong and hot. Someone who is cold and weak might benefit from this herb. However, anyone with a heat condition might get worse and end up with stressed adrenals, because Ginseng can increase *pitta*. American Ginseng (*Panax quinquefolium*) is somewhat cooler and gentler and can be useful in many cases. However, those with high *pitta* should use either of these forms of Ginseng with extreme care, if at all.

Siberian Ginseng (*Eleutherococcus senticosus*). Although not a true ginseng, Siberian Ginseng also works at a deep level to support immunity and adrenal function. It is much gentler and cooler than either Korean or American Ginseng and can be used by almost everyone. This herb can be taken over the long term for gentle support by anyone with immune dysfunction. Siberian Ginseng is acceptable for all *doshas* and can be taken safely by most *pittas*.

Astragalus (*Astragalus membranaceus*). Astragalus is an herb that has been used for thousands of years, first by the Chinese and now by western herbalists. It is a deep immune tonic that works slowly in the bone marrow. Astragalus helps the bone marrow to manufacture more white blood cells and to speed up their maturation rate. You need to use Astragalus for at least six to eight weeks before you begin to see any significant changes. Astragalus can be used by all three *doshas*.

Ashwagandha (*Withania somnifera*). Ashwagandha holds a place in Ayurvedic pharmacology similar to ginseng in Chinese medicine, yet it is far less expensive. It is an excellent rejuvenative herb and can be used in all conditions of weakness and tissue deficiency in children, the elderly, those debilitated by chronic diseases, and those suffering from overwork, lack of sleep or nervous exhaustion. Ashwagandha inhibits aging and catalyzes the anabolic processes of the body. It is an excellent herb for the mind, because it is nurturing and clarifying. It is calming and promotes deep, dreamless sleep. Although some herbalists feel that Ashwagandha is safe for pregnant women and helps to stabilize the fetus,[10] others question its use in pregnancy.

Ashwagandha is bitter, astringent and sweet, is heating, with a sweet post-digestive effect. It decreases *vata* and *kapha* and in excess may increase *pitta*.

Licorice (*Glycyrrhiza glabra*). Licorice is an effective adrenal tonic, and by strengthening the adrenals we also strengthen immunity. This herb is quite sweet and the powder makes a delicious tea, either alone or mixed with other herbs. Licorice is highly prized in Chinese Herbal Medicine and appears in almost every Chinese herbal formula. One word of caution about Licorice: If you have high blood pressure, don't overuse this herb, because in large quantities it tends to raise blood pressure by causing potassium loss and water retention.

Licorice is sweet and bitter, is cooling, with a sweet post-digestive effect. It decreases *vata* and *pitta*. It may increase *kapha* if taken long term.

Supplements for a Strong Immunity

In an ideal world, we would not need to take supplements. However, because of our depleted soil, stressful lifestyles and polluted environment, our immunity needs help. There are a few basic supplements we feel everyone should include, even apart from signs of imbalance. If specific problems are evident, see the chapter on treatment for additional suggestions.

Green Drinks. There are a number of green drinks available in natural food stores. They vary in quality, but many of them are delicious and of high quality. Read the labels and compare. Two good choices are Green Magic and Greens+. Margaret's favorite is Greens+, a green powder containing concentrated sources of organic vitamins, minerals, essential amino acids, and other important nutrients. Three teaspoons of this product in four ounces of juice or water each morning is a good way to start the day. Shoshana prefers the taste of Green Magic. A day without greens is a day that "sags" a bit. If you don't follow through on anything else suggested in this section, choose a high quality green drink and take it every day. These drinks are good for all three *doshas*. Sources are available in the Appendix.

Vitamin C. Next in importance is Vitamin C. It is almost impossible to eat enough food rich in Vitamin C, and supplementation is easy and enormously helpful and protective. Don't use ascorbic acid, because it can create an acidic condition in your body. Vitamin C as ascorbates is preferable and is easily utilized by the body, without side effects. How much should you take? That depends on your individual makeup and the level of stress in your life. Appropriate dosage can range from 500 mg per day up to 10 grams. Generally, 1000 to 2000 mg per day is the recommended amount.

If Vitamin C is taken as ascorbates on an empty stomach, it neutralizes acidity and removes *pitta* from the body. Vitamin C as ascorbic acid, taken with or after food, tends to build acidity and *pitta* in the body. If you choose an ascorbate form, Vitamin C is easily utilized by all *doshas*.

Flaxseed Oil and Seeds (*Cinum usitatissimum*). We have already discussed the value of flaxseed oil, and all of us need to include this valuable nutrient in our daily diets. Choose an oil from the refrigerated section of your natural food store (Barlean's is a good choice) and always keep it refrigerated. If it begins to smell or taste rancid, throw it out. Rancid oil can do more harm than good. It you find it difficult to take the oil in liquid form, it is also available in gel caps.

Another excellent way to include this nutrient is through its seeds. Most natural food stores sell whole flaxseeds. They are delicious and crunchy and can be used as ground nuts on cereals and other foods. Once flaxseeds are ground, they are as volatile as the oil and must be kept cold. Grind only as much as you are going to eat, or store them in the freezer.

Flaxseeds have been part of the human diet for at least 10,000 years. Hippocrates extolled their virtues, and the Greeks added flaxseed flour to their wheat flour when making bread. In Europe, flaxseeds still play a major role in the diet. The Germans, for example, consume 60,000 tons annually in breads and cereals. We eat so little in the United States that no one has bothered to measure our consumption. Mahatma Gandhi is credited with saying: "Wherever flaxseeds become a regular food item among the people, there will be better health."[11]

Flaxseeds are a good tonic for *vata*, for the colon and the lungs. They strengthen lung tissue and promote the healing of the lung membranes. They are also a good laxative for *vata*. Grind a spoonful and take before sleep for constipation, either straight or made into a warm infusion.[12]

Flaxseeds are sweet and astringent, heating, with a pungent post-digestive effect. They decrease *vata* and *pitta* and may increase *kapha*.

Multi-Vitamin/Mineral. We also feel that everyone should be on a good multi-vitamin/mineral supplement. There are many good products available in natural food stores. Although a green drink goes a long way toward providing necessary nutrients, we still feel adding a good quality multi-vitamin/mineral supplement is necessary in today's world. We also recommend additional supplementation of calcium and magnesium.

A word about calcium: The most common form of calcium found in supplements is calcium carbonate, which is nothing but chalk and difficult for the body to absorb. Read the label on your supplement bottle. Any other form of calcium is better—citrate, malate, fumarate or ascorbate—and much more absorbable.

Incidentally, if you take Tums for calcium, there are better sources. The calcium in Tums is calcium carbonate, which can only be absorbed by the body in the presence of hydrochloric acid. Taking calcium along with an antacid (which neutralizes hydrochloric acid) sets up a body chemistry in which absorption of the calcium is impossible.

We all too often pop Tums or other antacids into our mouths at the first sign of stomach pain. However, many times the pain is due to a *low* level of hydrochloric acid rather than a *high* one, and we only increase the problem by taking an antacid substance. Often what is really needed for this condition is something to *boost* the hydrochloric acid. Low acidity, called hypochlorhydria, can develop into a serious condition, including cancer, if it remains for a long time. Therefore, anything like Tums that lowers an already low acidity is to be avoided. As we age, problems with low stomach acidity become quite common.

Magnesium is also a vital mineral. It is widely accepted at this point that magnesium should be taken in equal ratio to calcium, rather than in a ratio of two parts calcium to one part magnesium, as has been practiced in recent years. Again, read your label.

CHAPTER **13**

TIPS FOR TRAVEL: WHAT TO TAKE WITH YOU[1]

WE'VE TALKED ABOUT HERBS and other ways to stay in balance when you are at home. Now let's switch our attention to the important question of meeting health challenges when you are away from home. Travel can be fun and rewarding. However, falling ill when away from home can turn your trip into a nightmare.

One of the secrets to good health on a trip is taking care of yourself before you leave home. Proper rest and herbs to boost your immunity in preparation for a trip are good investments. In addition, carrying with you some carefully chosen items can help ensure restoring balance if you have an upset. Let's have a look at some substances that might be useful. Everything discussed here is safe for children—except for aspirin—and can be used in modified dosages according to the age of the child.

How well prepared you need to be depends on where you are going and what you will have available while away from home. If you are travelling to a tropical country and will basically be on your own, you must be much more prepared than on a cruise complete with medical facilities. However, no matter where your travels take you, there are some basic items for self care that are quite useful. In fact, just having a kit of these substances in your car for short trips is also a good idea.

Activated Charcoal. This substance is placed at the top of the list because of its usefulness in many conditions. Activated charcoal *adsorbs*, gathers to itself, up to 17 times its weight of whatever surrounds it. This form of charcoal is made by burning vegetable material and then treating the carbon residue to increase its adsorptive surface. The process of *absorption* is slow and involves substances crossing cell membranes. *Adsorption* is a mechanical process that happens quickly and the substances involved, such as activated charcoal, act like chemical sponges.

Buy activated charcoal in capsule form. If you experience a topical infection of any kind or a venomous bite or sting—even a snake bite—open several caps, moisten the charcoal, place the moistened charcoal on a clean cloth or bandage and apply to the wound. The charcoal will draw off the poison. You might want to use a paper cup or some container you can throw away for moistening the charcoal, because the charcoal will discolor the container.

For internal poisoning from food or other substances, take three or four caps internally. The charcoal will *adsorb* the poison and pass it out of the body. Activated charcoal can also be used for diarrhea. If there is no relief from the diarrhea in three to four hours, take another dose of three to four caps. Yes, it can be constipating. However, deal with the diarrhea first, because diarrhea can lead to dehydration and serious problems.

Aspirin. This substance, so common to us these days, was originally derived from Willow Bark (*Salix sp.*). It is anti-inflammatory, antipyretic (lowers fever), analgesic (eases pain) and decreases platelet aggravation (decreases risk of blood clotting). Don't give aspirin to children, because of its association with the development of Reye's Syndrome.

Aspirin is the drug of choice if someone is having an embolic stroke, a stroke involving a blood clot, because of its action on clotting. Most strokes are caused by clots, rather than by hemorrhages. Alka Seltzer is a form of aspirin that works quickly and can be safely used if there is no elevation in blood pressure. The sodium bicarbonate in the Alka Seltzer buffers the gastric irritating effect of pure aspirin.

Aspirin is a good anti-inflammatory and is the antipyretic (fever lowering) substance of choice for adults. Children can tolerate a much higher fever than adults. If a child has a fever over 104 degrees, give a neutral temperature bath to lower the fever.

Bromelain. Bromelain is a sulfur containing substance from the stem of the pineapple plant. It can be used for all types of inflammation and infection. It works well or better than antibiotics for sinusitis, because of its mucous dissolving action. Use at the first sign of colds or flus to avoid development of any bacterial or other secondary infection. The capsule form is faster acting than the pill form.

Bromelain is also helpful in sprains, strains and wound healing. It helps to clear out the products of inflammation and speeds the healing process.

Take one or two caps three or four times a day *between* meals for action against infection. If Bromalain is taken *with* food, it will aid digestion but will have no anti-infective action.

Echinacea and Goldenseal (*E. angustifolia* or *E. purpurea* and *Hydrastis canadensis*). Echinacea is a "must have" herb when traveling. For several days before leaving on a plane trip, take one-half teaspoon of Echinacea tincture three times a day to boost your immunity. Continue this dosage for a few days after arrival. Breathing the dry and recycled air aboard a plane can be a challenge at the beginning of a trip.

Be sure you have a potent tincture of Echinacea. If the tincture doesn't "bite" your tongue, temporarily leaving a slightly numb feeling, try another brand. In addition, when dosing yourself, be sure to take enough. This herb is quite safe for adults and children. If you want to avoid an alcohol tincture for a child, buy one that has been prepared with vegetable glycerine.

In addition to Echinacea in preparation for a trip, it is wise to take a deep immune stimulant, such as Astragalus or Siberian Ginseng, for several weeks or months. These herbs work slowly and must be taken over a long period of time to reap their benefits. High quality tinctures or tablets are available. In contrast, Echinacea works quickly for acute conditions.

Goldenseal is a threatened species and should not be used unless there is no substitute. However, when traveling it is wise to have some of it along. A combination of Echinacea and Goldenseal provides a broad spectrum antibiotic that fights bacteria, viruses and fungi. And it is safe to use with children. Check out the Goldenseal you buy to be sure it was not wildcrafted. Many herb companies are now growing their own Goldenseal, so be sure you buy one of those labels.

Some herbalists feel that Goldenseal is contraindicated in pregnancy. If you are pregnant, Echinacea is a safe alternative.

Start taking Echinacea and Goldenseal—one-half to one teaspoon three times a day—at the first sign of an infection of any kind, whether it is bacterial or viral. Be sure to take enough. If you don't get results, you haven't dosed heavily enough. Continue taking the treatment until symptoms are gone, for one to two weeks.

A combination tincture of Echinacea and Goldenseal can also be used topically on wounds or bites as a powerful disinfectant. Taking herbs along in tincture form increases the range of their usefulness.

Ginkgo (*Ginkgo biloba*). If a trip is quite long and involves hours of sitting, Ginkgo can be useful to keep the circulation moving. This herb is a stimulant to peripheral circulation. Begin taking small doses of Ginkgo a few days before traveling. A day or two before a long plane trip, for example, increase the dose to 80 milligrams three times a day. If you experience no headache or gastrointestinal upset from that amount, you may want to increase the dose. After arrival, decrease the dose gradually. Ginkgo is quite safe. Because of Ginkgo's ability to inhibit platelet aggregation, care should probably be taken if you are on a drug such as Cumadin or other blood thinners.

In addition to Ginkgo, when on a long plane trip, don't forget to twist and turn your ankles and move about as much as possible. If you have an airport wait, get down on the floor and do some stretching, which will help to keep your circulation moving.

Relaxing Herbs. Traveling can be stressful and sleep may be difficult. In addition to Melatonin, which will be discussed for helping to reset your internal clock, you might want to try Kava Kava (*Piper methysticum*), Valerian (*Valeriana officinalis*), or Skullcap (*Scutellaria lateriflora*). Experiment with these herbs ahead of time, so you know what works for you. A relaxing tea such as Chamomile is also useful. These herbs are quite calming for *vata*.

Peppermint (*Mentha piperata*). Peppermint tea helps to calm an upset gastrointestinal tract. Use for nausea, vomiting or colicky bowel gas. Enteric coated capsules of peppermint are helpful in cases of irritable bowel syndrome or spasm. Peppermint reduces gastric secretion (acidity) and increases stomach emptying speed by over 40 percent. These effects are ideal for simple overindulgence. Peppermint is cooling for *pitta*.

Chamomile (*Matricaria chamomila*). Make a strong tea of chamomile and use it for colitis, intestinal spasm, colic or respiratory infection. For food poisoning make a strong tea of chamomile and peppermint. For inflammation on the skin, place a wet teabag directly on the inflammation. If the skin is inflamed over a large area, try a bath of chamomile tea. Placing a wet teabag over an inflamed eye can also be helpful. Chamomile is also a mild nervine and helps calm anxiety and restlessness. A cup of chamomile tea before sleep is sometimes quite helpful. Chamomile is calming for *vata*.

Cayenne (*Capsicum sp.*). Cayenne is a powerful circulatory stimulant. In case of shock, or even heart attack, place a few drops of Cayenne tincture under the tongue. Repeat, if necessary. This strong stimulant will usually bring a person around. If you don't have cayenne available in an emergency, Tobasco can be used instead. You have experienced the increased circulatory action of Cayenne if you have eaten hot salsa in a Mexican restaurant. Your face breaks out in a sweat and your heart beats faster.

For bleeding, apply Cayenne externally. A tincture of Cayenne can be applied directly to a wound. Initially it will burn due to the release of Substance P. However, once Substance P has been fully released, the pain will disappear.

Another way of using Cayenne externally is to make a cream by adding Cayenne powder to your favorite body cream. This cream can be rubbed on areas of neuralgia pain. Again, once Substance P is fully released, the pain will disappear.

A few drops of Cayenne tincture under the tongue is a good treatment for cluster or migraine headaches. Your tincture must be powerful and it will burn. (According to Dana Myatt, ND, a high quality tincture will raise the dead. And, if it doesn't, the person is indeed dead!)

Cayenne is an extremely hot substance and must be used carefully by people with hot constitutions (*pittas*). However, in cases of shock, heart attack, bleeding, severe pain of headache and neuralgia, this substance in tincture or cream form can be lifesaving, even for *pittas*!

Castor Oil (*Palma Christi*). Castor oil has mild steroid action and can be used externally for many kinds of pain, including pain associated with gallbladder problems, kidney stones, cystitis, menses, hepatitis, systemic infections or musculo-skeletal problems. The actions of castor oil are antispasmodic, analgesic and immunomodulating.

Almost everyone who has heard of Edgar Cayce has heard of his extensive use of castor oil packs. While the medicinal properties of the oil of the castor bean have been known for thousands of years, Cayce's use of castor oil in packs seems to have been distinctively his.

To prepare a castor oil pack, take three to four thicknesses of clean cloth, preferably unbleached white wool flannel, and saturate the cloth with castor oil, which is hexane free—available in all natural food stores. Heat this pack in an oven, or place it directly over the site of pain and cover with a heating pad. Protect the bed or surrounding area with a plastic covering. Keep the pack on the area of pain for about an hour. Repeat once a day for several days, depending on the severity of the pain. The oil soaked cloth can be stored in a plastic bag for reuse.[2] Don't use a castor oil pack if appendicitis is suspected. The heat applied to the pack might aggravate the condition.

Tea Tree Oil (*Melaleuca alternifolia*). Tea tree oil excels as a potent antiseptic and is a "pharmacy" in a tiny bottle. It can also be used for athlete's foot and other fungal conditions. A drop of the oil in a small amount of water swished in the mouth is good for irritations. Also use a dilution of the oil to brush the teeth and massage the gums. Don't take the oil internally.

Arnica Cream and Tiger Balm. For sore bruises or strains, rub on Arnica cream. For sore muscles and joints, the warming effect of Tiger Balm is quite helpful.

Ginger (*Zingibar officinale*). Ginger is a must in the travel kit, especially if you are prone to motion sickness. Buy in capsules or fill OO caps with dried ginger powder, and take two of the caps before getting on a plane. Take dried ginger powder with you for use as a tea for any type of stomach complaint. A small bottle of alcohol tincture of ginger also has many uses. Add a few drops to tea or to your food for a bit of "zing." A tincture can also be taken directly into the mouth and will be immediately utilized by the body for altitude sickness or nausea. Ginger is also helpful for jet lag. Although ginger is a highly beneficial medicine, it is a hot substance. If you have a hot constitution *(pitta)*, be aware that excessive use may aggravate a hot condition. Try peppermint instead, which is cooling.

Melatonin. For traveling over several time zones and resulting jet lag, melatonin can be useful in helping to reset your biological clock. Try the sublingual tablets from Source Naturals, widely available in natural food stores.

Rescue Remedy. If you find yourself in a stressful situation, or if you have experienced a bite or sting which creates stress, a few drops of Rescue Remedy can help to bring relaxation. In a case of shock, place a few drops on the lips or under the tongue.

Bitters. Bitter is good for the liver and you can help protect yourself from all kinds of parasites by including the bitter taste in your diet. An easily available source is Angostura Aromatic Bitters, available at any liquor store. This product is made from the Chinese herb Gentian (*Gentiana lutea*), considered in Chinese Herbal Medicine to be an important herb for the liver. Take a sip a day to keep the bugs away. If the bugs get hold, increase the dose. Bitters are cooling and act on *pitta*.

Another readily available herb for the liver is Milk Thistle (*Silybum marianum*). This herb will help protect the liver and is a good choice to include at home or while traveling.

Yogurt. Yogurt is widely available in many parts of the world, and eating it daily is an easy way to keep the "good bacteria" in control of your colon. In fact, eating a small amount twice daily is a good practice. If you are traveling in India (or elsewhere), try a glass of *lassi* each day. See page 210 for a recipe.

Constipation. Many people experience constipation while traveling. Include in your kit some form of fiber, such as psyllium husks (widely available as Metamucil), and as a precaution be sure to eat plenty of fiber in your daily diet.

Additional Suggestions. One of the most useful travel companions that one can have—whether the trip is long or short—is a supply of 2" by

2" individually wrapped wipes. These wipes are useful not only to clean your hands but can also be used to clean questionable silverware, a dirty knife, or even as toilet paper in a pinch.

A suggestion for stopping bleeding: A plain ordinary wet teabag of black tea is quite astringent. Place the wet bag directly over the site of bleeding. And don't forget to include Band-Aids in a variety of sizes for minor cuts and scratches.

In locations where air pollution is particularly bad, a mixture of one-third turmeric powder and two-thirds mineral or sea salt makes a soothing gargle. Take the mixture along in powdered form and mix with water as needed. The powerful antibiotic action of this mixture can help ward off bugs that might cause a sore throat or worse to develop.

Since the quality of drinking water is questionable in many areas, having some water purification tablets with you may be helpful. They are available in stores that sell camping and outdoor equipment.

Finally, pack a long, wide, lightweight cotton scarf, which can be easily washed. The scarf can be used as a cover for questionable bedding, as a pillow, as a light blanket, or a filter to breathe through when the air is full of particles and pollution. It can also be used as an arm sling if needed.

General Guidelines for Healthy and Happy Traveling.
- Get adequate rest.
- Invest time in personal hygiene. Keep even minor wounds clean. Wash hands with soap and water and keep clothes and bedding clean.
- Drink plenty of liquids. Dehydration can be a problem, especially in hot climates. Boil your water for drinking or purchase bottled water. Avoid ice cubes. If you can't find pure water, add two drops of bleach per cup or a water purification tablet. Small filtration units are also available in outdoor and camping stores.
- Eat carefully chosen food and keep overindulgence to a minimum.
- If in a tropical country, protect yourself with mosquito netting while sleeping.
- Use sunblock, sunglasses and a hat.
- Protect your feet. Keep them clean and dry and do not go barefoot. If you develop a blister or skin break, treat it immediately and protect the area.
- Eat only cooked food, unless you are in an area you know is safe.

* * * * *

Choose from the many suggestions here, depending on where you are going and what works for you. The amount of each item you take will depend on how long you will be away. Be sure to take an adequate supply of Echinacea and Goldenseal, which can be combined if you wish. Four ounces is probably a minimum amount. On the other hand, one-half ounce of Cayenne is probably adequate.

While traveling, as well as at home, it is important to eat well, get adequate rest, exercise often, and maintain a healthy and positive outlook. Remember that the mind-body connection is strong, and worrying about your health will probably weaken your immunity. Go prepared with your travel kit, follow a healthy lifestyle, and have fun.

Items to Pack	
Activated Charcoal Capsules	• Internal poisoning from food or other substance • Diarrhea • Venomous bites or stings
Bromelain Capsules	• Inflammation and infection • Dissolves mucus • Sprains, strains and wound healing • Digestive aid
Aspirin	• Reduces inflammation • Lowers fever • Eases pain • Decreases risk of blood clotting
Echinacea Tincture Goldenseal Tincture	• Antibiotic and antiviral for acute conditions • Topical disinfectant for wounds and bites
Ginkgo	• Circulatory stimulant
Peppermint Tea Bags	• Calms gastrointestinal tract • Nausea, vomiting, gas • Irritable bowel syndrome or spasm • Reduces gastric acidity • Increases stomach emptying speed

Chamomile Tea Bags	• Colitis • Intestinal spasm • Respiratory infection • Skin inflammation • Calm anxiety and restlessness
Cayenne Tincture	• Circulatory stimulant • Shock • Heart attack • External bleeding • Neuralgia pain in cream form • Cluster or migraine headaches
Castor Oil	• Mild steroid action • Apply externally as a pack for pain from gallbladder, kidney stones, cystitis, menses, hepatitis, systemic infection, musculo-skeletal problems
Tea Tree Oil	• Antiseptic • Anti-fungal • Anti-inflammatory
Arnica Cream Tiger Balm	• Sore bruises or strains • Sore muscles and joints
Ginger Powder	• Motion sickness • Stomach upset • Jet lag
Melatonin Tablets	• Sleep aid • Reset biological clock
Rescue Remedy	• Stress • Shock
Bitters Milk Thistle	• Protection from parasites • Protection of liver
Psyllium Husks or Metamucil	• Constipation
Turmeric Powder and Salt for Gargle	• Antibiotic action • As gargle protects throat
Individually Wrapped Wipes	• Multiple uses
BandAids	• Minor cuts and scratches
Large Cotton Scarf	• Multiple uses

Medicine of the Twenty-first Century: A New Paradigm That Moves Beyond the Physical

"The significant problems we have cannot be solved at the same level of thinking with which we created them."

—Albert Einstein

THROUGHOUT THIS BOOK the focus has been one of self-help. Looking at yourself in the ways we have developed enables you to understand the location(s) of any imbalances which cause you difficulty. Your observations should provide you with all the "clues" you need, and the Eastern concepts of the characteristics associated with the *doshas*—*vata, pitta* and *kapha*—should enable you to know what route or routes to take to re-establish balance.

The thrust of this book has been on the practical. You can get a sense of how great an imbalance is by simply counting the number of locations that indicate a similar imbalance. The locations are the face, tongue, hands and nails, ears, eyes, feet and meridians. The more locations, the greater the imbalance. When there are many imbalances of different kinds, you need not become overwhelmed or discouraged. You should simply check the symptoms against the qualities of *vata, pitta* and *kapha* and work on one *dosha* at a time. Multiple symptoms may all have one common *doshic* source. You can have four things in an oven at one time and they can all be burning. Each item can be analyzed separately to determine the degree of burning, etc. But if you want to prevent additional burning, just turn down the oven temperature. So it is with *pitta* heat. Similarly, reduction in the qualities associated with each *dosha* reduces the imbalances inherent in that *dosha*. Reduce the cool, dry qualities of *vata* or the dense, congesting qualities of *kapha,* and all related symptoms decrease.

The system we have outlined is both simple and profound. Many of the concepts are now being scientifically validated here in the West and are changing the way we look at health and the way medicine is practiced. Indeed, a huge paradigm shift is currently underway. The shift is changing our ideas about the very basis of reality, moving away from a mechanistic, deterministic view focused solely on the body, to a view that affirms the dynamism of our being, that relates body, mind and consciousness to constantly changing flows of transformative energies interacting with physical matter.

We submit that the paradigm shift currently under way brings us close to the basic concepts of Dynamic Ayurveda. Indeed, what we are beginning to discover is that ancient concepts are re-emerging and forming the foundation of a new scientific medical model. The remainder of this chapter identifies some of these ancient concepts present and reflected in modern scientific research, research that is beginning to transform the way medicine is practiced.

The Paradigm Shift

Out of the ashes of every major era there is transformative change. Change comes not only from the decay of previous ideas, values and outdated systems, but also from emerging views of a different reality. We are currently in the midst of a medical paradigm shift. We believe that ultimately the new paradigm will be based on a blending of Eastern and Western approaches to medicine, utilizing information garnered from the human genome project, to better understand the relationship between genetic predisposition (what we call constitution) and current lifestyle to understand the physical part of disease, and utilizing Eastern concepts to understand how those physical aspects are influenced by mind and consciousness and the *doshas*. With the passage of time, we believe that the most dynamic aspects of Ayurveda will be validated by scientific research. This blend of scientific research and Ayurvedic concepts can be viewed as a modern 21st century form which we call Dynamic Ayurveda.

Dynamic Ayurveda

In this book we have studied much that has come to us from ancient times. What makes this knowledge relevant to us today? That which is true and vital has a dynamism that is timeless. Although the people who developed this knowledge thousands of years ago had no scientific methods of "proving" the validity of their approach, we will review some of the scientific research that parallels these ancient truths. Many of the scientific studies which purport to advance "new understanding" about human health and disease are restating in modern language ancient concepts that have worked well for thousands of years.

The paradigm shift that is taking place all around us is built on the following foundations:

- **You are more than the sum-total of your physical parts. You are also an energy system composed of mind and consciousness as well as body.**
- **What happens to your body is never an arbitrary development. There is an intimate relationship between how you use your energy, how your energy flows within your physical systems and the development of the disease process.**
- **You can develop self-understanding by becoming aware of the way basic qualities are affecting you. These qualities are associated with the energy balances/imbalances of *vata, pitta* and *kapha*. The qualities are pairs of opposites: hot-cold, rough-smooth, sharp-dull, dry-wet, heavy-light, hard-soft, etc. These qualities are reflected in every element of your being—consciousness, mind, emotions, intellect, body.**
- **Qualities are not fixed. You can increase or decrease any quality at any level of your being. Like quality increases, opposite quality decreases.**
- **Personal attention to your thought patterns and beliefs plays a key role in what happens to you. In the absence of personal attention, you are a victim of your unconscious beliefs and behaviors. As you become aware of personal thought patterns, you begin to gain conscious control over them.**

- It is possible to reprogram your beliefs—both conscious and unconscious—by developing your creative/intuitive capabilities, by vividly infusing new beliefs with your attention, and by acting in line with these beliefs. Both the conscious and unconscious mind will respond. You can foster this process in many ways, all of which initially involve quieting the ramblings in your mind. Some of the "tools" you can use are diet, herbs and supplements, exercise, relaxation techniques, yoga, meditation. Symbols, colors, sounds (including music), light and space can also be used to support subtle changes.
- With focused attention you can become aware of resistances and, moving beyond rationalizations, can slowly but surely remove your own internal obstacles to creating a healthier, happier life.

In the process of gaining new levels of control over your health and your life, you will discover changes in your concept of personal responsibility. It will no longer be enough to observe that you feel ill and should visit a doctor. You will not be content to merely swallow medications or undergo surgeries. In understanding the disease process and your role in fostering or curtailing that process, you will have greater choices in reacting.

Centuries ago there was a decline of authority. The authority of the church was questioned and this led to a separation of church and state. Now the authority of the state and business is being questioned. The authority of the expert is also being questioned. Instead of thinking "How can THEY (the experts, the government, big business, the doctor— whoever) take care of us?" the question now is "How can THEY support us, and help us figure out for ourselves what we want to do?" Everywhere you look you can observe people wanting to take responsibility for their decisions while having institutions support them by providing information and services to help them move forward. We no longer trust others to look out for our welfare. This means that the individual is conceptually being placed in a position of control.

The notion that "I am responsible for myself" means we must learn the vital connections between body, mind and consciousness in order to function adequately in the world. We must move from concepts of victimization, where someone else or something else is responsible for the bad things that happen to us, to an awareness of the part we play in creating our realities, and then from there we can move on to even higher levels of awareness, fostering inner harmonies compatible with our own notions of the universal life force, by whatever name it might be called.

With fresh awareness comes multiple ways of increasing knowledge. The scientific emphasis on research is being expanded from rigid, physically oriented studies to ones which include the ways attention and intuition affect our knowledge and behavior.

In both Ayurveda and Chinese medicine there is a saying that the microcosm reflects the macrocosm. On a personal level you can become aware that all your cells have "intelligence." They are in the process of communication all the time, are involved in the relationship of matter and "you," and link you to the "universe," the world outside you. This concept has been part of Ayurveda for thousands of years but has only recently found its way into Western scientific thinking.

Dynamic Ayurveda as Reflected in Modern Scientific Research

We list ten concepts of Dynamic Ayurveda that have scientific support.

1. Body, mind and consciousness are inseparable and cannot be compartmentalized.
2. That which affects the body also affects the mind and consciousness and vice versa.
3. There is intelligence in all the cells of the body.
4. The cells communicate with one another.
5. People have different constitutions that make them susceptible to different illnesses. Our lifestyles—diet, exercise, environment, emotions and belief systems—profoundly affect our health.
6. Disease can result from a combination of genetic (*doshic*) susceptibility and our total inner and outer environment.

7. Mind and consciousness work through the body but are not contained within it.
8. Mind and consciousness can bring us to states of awareness that enhance our health.
9. The life force exists within us and around us and we can readily tap into it with intention and attention.
10. The world of the mind is expansive and not contained by the current limited view of reality.

Significant research has been done in leading scientific institutions throughout the world that supports these almost mind-boggling concepts. Recent work in decoding DNA and the resulting information about our genomic makeup leads us away from a mechanistic view of the body to one that sees the body as a complex information system. It is now recognized that cells are coded with information and can communicate with other cells, indeed that they have a certain level of "intelligence." Electricity flows through our brains, and chemicals in our brains pick up electrical signals and send coded information that tells our cells what to do. "DNA, proteins and all the precisely sculptured molecules of the biological world are thus charged with information."[1] Electrical impulses transport information bits that allow communication within cells and between cells. This is a profoundly different way of viewing the body. No longer can we treat it as a simple biochemical system. Instead it is now clear that there is a profound relationship between the physical and electromagnetic energy, between matter and energy.

A new approach to medicine is emerging called *functional medicine*. Dr. Jeffrey Bland at the Institute for Functional Medicine in Gig Harbor, Washington, is one of the leaders in this new field. Functional medicine is defined as a field of healthcare that employs assessment and early intervention before the onset of diagnosable disease to improve physiological, emotional/cognitive and physical function. Using a wide range of academic and clinical disciplines, it treats illness and promotes vitality by focusing on the root levels of metabolic imbalance. Rather than merely suppressing symptoms without treating the actual cause of the disease process, functional medicine aims to improve and optimize health at the psychological, biochemical or structural levels through therapies that restore, repair and rebuild balance. This is Dynamic Ayurveda, a modern statement of ancient truths. The approach of functional medicine parallels the first three stages of the Ayurvedic process of disease, as discussed in Chapter Seven.

Functional medicine emphasizes the importance of treating the individual rather than merely the disease. Disease classification then is not as important as identifying the cause at the genetic-molecular-environmental level. Assessment is concerned with understanding the antecedents, triggers and mediators of dysfunction that give rise to imbalances underlying the signs and symptoms of disease. Fundamental to functional medicine is an awareness of the web-like interactions of all systems. For example, in functional medicine as in Eastern medicine, a cancerous tumor is viewed as more than a tumor—it is an expression of imbalance throughout the body.

The Institute for Functional Medicine is performing and compiling scientific research that supports this new approach to healthcare. It will take a number of years for this information to be incorporated into widespread medical practice. However, this new approach holds promise for the future and will greatly enhance prediction and prevention of disease.

A number of labs across the country have developed functional assessment tests to assist in identifying early stages of imbalance. These tests are valuable tools for the practitioner. Contact information for several of these labs is included in the Resources appendix.

Eastern medicine, and Ayurveda in particular, considers the body/mind/consciousness connection as basic. In fact, in Ayurveda there is no perceived separation, no border, separating these three. Dr. Vasant Lad, our Ayurvedic teacher, speaks of the crystallization of emotions, the process by which unresolved emotions become actual physical substances lodged in our tissues. Dr. Candace Pert, a psychoneuroimmunologist formerly with the National Institute of Mental Health, now at Georgetown University, upholds this view and maintains that emotions have a physical component that affects the biochemical processes of the body. Dr. Pert and her husband collegue Dr. Michael Ruff have conducted leading edge research documenting these insights. See her book *Molecules of Emotion*. They have discovered the amazing influence that emotions have on the functioning of peptides on cellular receptors. This discovery is particularly significant because it demonstrates that cells have intelligence and communicate information to other cells. The cells of diverse systems, such as the nervous, immune, digestive and reproductive systems, communicate with one another. One's emotional state profoundly affects the functioning of these communicating peptides, directly linking the body and mind into one holistic system. Within this linkage the mind can either introduce toxins into the cells or play an important role in their detoxification. This process is a two way street: the amount of toxins in the cells can also affect the mind. The interplay is constant between the two. Hence, high emotional stress can lead to physical imbalances, symptoms and diseases—and vice versa. As in Ayurveda, Dr. Pert recognizes that techniques such as meditation, visualization, dream work and energy work can have a measurable and profound effect on calming the mind and healing the body/mind/consciousness connection.[2]

Dr. Larry Dossey maintains that the mind is not contained within the body and is not limited by time and space. Citing the work of scientists at such institutions as Princeton, Harvard and Stanford, he makes the case that spiritual tools such as intercessory prayer, dreams, and intuition have measurable, powerful and profound effects on how we heal, and influence us in ways we do not yet understand scientifically. Intention and attention impact the healing of wounds.[3]

Dr. Dossey cites scientific evidence showing that the healing process is profoundly affected by "nonlocal" healing, energy projections from other sources. Focused awareness of positive, loving thoughts can be projected to others in ways that positively affect the healing process. Dr. Dossey suggests that nonlocal mind can affect diagnosis and treatment of disease. We call this consciousness, and we use consciousness in our own practices, often with amazing results.[4]

Fascinating research and clinical work is being done by Carolyn McMakin on the effects of low frequency microcurrent stimulation on a wide range of chronic illnesses for which there are few if any effective treatments. This form of stimulation is particularly effective for myofascial pain, fibromyalgia, nerve root irritation, tendon and ligament repair and pain related to acute trauma.

Carolyn McMakin's pioneering work with chronic pain hypothesizes that each organ and tissue of the body has an electrical frequency, a vibrational pattern, that is unique to that organ or tissue. When injury occurs, the pattern is altered. Low frequency microcurrent treatment can help reestablish normal frequencies in injured cells. In cases of trauma, for example, inflammation usually occurs. After as little as 20 minutes of microcurrent treatment to injured areas, preliminary blood samples show positive changes in actual blood chemistry by reducing inflammatories and increasing anti-inflammatories. This is an area where we can expect further research and writing. Microcurrent appears to provide a helpful way to use technology in a non-invasive approach to pain.[5] It addition, it may well provide a method to apply the Eastern concepts of energy flow and meridians in practical ways without healthcare practitioners having to become expert in acupuncture or Ayurveda. Biopsy studies will give a better view of exactly how the microcurrent process works, but the clinical application of microcurrent has yielded impressive results in over 12,000 known applications. This is exciting work. Shoshana has incorporated microcurrent into her work.

The ability of scientific research to demonstrate the way emotions and the mind affect the physical is not only remarkable, it also implies that the nature of reality is far less physical than previously thought. Now work is being done on an even more subtle level: People are learning techniques to access and utilize basic life force energy to accelerate healing. The results can be and have been documented in the work of such people as Larry Dossey and Candance Pert. The idea that "laying on of hands" and "channeling of energy" can facilitate healing is not new. It is the scientific documentation of this process that is new.

Richard Gordon in *Quantum Touch*[6] describes this process, a process he has taught to thousands. He has taught workshops in medical schools and has introduced the approach to people such as Dr. C. Norman Shealy, the co-founder of the American Holistic Medical Association and a research and clinical professor of psychology. Gordon reports that Dr. Shealy and his staff use the technique with remarkable results on chronically ill individuals who often suffer from debilitating pain. Gordon is interested in exploring how consciousness and matter interact at the quantum, subatomic level.[7]

In recent years, Dr. Dean Ornish's work in reversing and treating heart disease has been well established. In addition to the profound impact exercise, diet, meditation and group support have on reversing heart disease, Dr. Ornish has discovered that love and intimacy are also powerful healers. In *Love and Survival*[8] Dr. Ornish persuasively argues that love and intimacy are at the root of what makes us sick and what makes us well, what causes sadness and what brings happiness, what makes us suffer and what leads to healing. He maintains that the real epidemic in our culture is not physical heart disease but emotional and spiritual heart disease—the profound sense of loneliness, isolation, alienation and depression that are so prevalent among us. Like Dr. Pert, Dr. Ornish maintains that emotions manifest in our bodies and can be a root cause of serious physical illness. This same concept, now viewed from a Western scientific perspective, has been advanced by Ayurveda for thousands of years. Ornish's views match those of Dynamic Ayurveda.

Others have offered insights into the body/mind/consciousness connection. Dr. Christiane Northrup's book *Women's Bodies, Women's Wisdom*[9] speaks of the magnificent way our very essence, our life force, is expressed at all levels. She links mental and emotional patterns to the ancient *chakra* system, pointing to areas of the body that hold unresolved emotion. Not only does Dr. Northrup discuss problems related to menstrual cycles, childbirth, fibroids, breast anatomy, etc., from the perspective of Western medicine, she also demonstrates that women who make healthy lifestyle changes heal faster, more completely and have fewer medical interventions.[10]

Caroline Myss in her book *Anatomy of the Spirit*[11] develops the *chakra* information into an understandable system that explains the links between the ways we use our life force energy, the *chakras*, and the energy consequences of belief patterns. Dr. Myss is a healer who explains in clear, concise language ways to use spiritual awareness and intention to facilitate self-understanding and healing. In a parallel way, Dr. Candace Pert has shown that the *chakras*, energy centers that link subtle energies to the physical body, correspond to the location of nerve bundles on each side of the spinal cord that are rich in information carrying peptides.[12]

The implications of insights such as these are profound. It means that we are on the edge of discovering how matter and energy interact on subtle levels to create our individual realities.

Dr. Deepak Chopra has been a leader in advancing the concept of body/mind/consciousness in his many books. His work is a modern expression of Ayurvedic concepts in Western terms. He does a magnificent job outlining the relationship between perception and reality. We have attempted to pick up where he leaves off, providing practical ways for you to use Ayurvedic concepts to understand what is happening in your body and to be able to take corrective actions to enhance your health and state of being.

Most of the creative work in scientific research mentioned above is a development of the 1990s when interest in "alternative medicine" came into national consciousness through the groundbreaking work of Bill Moyers. He was the first to bring national televised attention to the work of the pioneers in the field of the body/mind connection with his PBS series and book *Healing and the Mind*.[13] His interviews with Dean Ornish, Candace Pert, David Eisenberg, Jon Kabat-Zin, Naomi Remen and others explored the power of this approach.

There are many others who have contributed to the shifting paradigm, including Drs. Andrew Weil, Bernie Siegel and Herbert Benson. Each has brought insights that help us move away from a mechanistic approach to health to a holistic way. We are grateful to all of these trailblazers.

The Journey from the Outer to the Inner

Medicine in the 21st century is moving from a limited view of the mechanical and chemical interactions in the body, to a broader awareness of body, mind and consciousness. As we learn to tap into our basic life force, our *chi* or *prana,* and use it for healing purposes, we will have new ways of dealing with health that can be controlled by individuals rather than institutions. When the relationship between our genes and *doshas* becomes common knowledge, and when approaches to medicine take into account the total person—body, mind and consciousness—as well as one's relationship to the external world, it will become possible for people to truly manage their health in ways we cannot even imagine at this time.

Why do you feel so bad when you have been declared perfectly healthy? In this book we attempted to provide you with the tools to answer this question for yourself. The concepts that we have presented about energy flow in the form of *vata, pitta* and *kapha* describe the process of disease, offer ancient diagnostic tools to understand energy imbalances, and provide many alternative ways of bringing oneself into balance. Gaining balance can rejuvenate you while simultaneously strengthening your immune system. With awareness of your own healthcare concerns, you can use the information we have provided in many ways.

What we have attempted in this book is to provide you with useful "tools" to help you analyze and correct your imbalances. Our approach has been to emphasize the most obvious impacts that diet, exercise and relaxation techniques can have on your health. However, we have only scratched the surface, for we have not explored more subtle influences. Essentially we are affected by anything that influences the senses. Hence problems can be approached from many directions. Color, touch, aroma and sound affect us in profound ways, a fact understood by advertisers, movie makers, musicians and other entertainers better than by physicians.

In addition to our senses, we are all affected by the strength or weakness, clarity or dullness of our emotions and awareness from moment to moment. The relationship between conscious awareness, emotions and our physical bodies is a new frontier for exploration.

Of the many recommendations made in this book, explore those that make sense to you and incorporate them into your life, starting with the changes that are easiest for you. Move slowly and gradually at your own pace. Set your own goals. For many it will be enough simply to become free of pain or to have enough energy to enjoy life more. For others, goals may be more ambitious. For those, we have attempted to provide new ideas, or old ideas from fresh perspectives, that can lead to giant steps forward to a healthy, exciting and deeply meaningful life.

We are indeed in the midst of an exciting medical paradigm shift. It is truly an exciting time to be alive! Self-healing is a highly individual process and requires reestablishing harmony within yourself and among all parts of yourself. Commit to developing the best that is within you, to living your dreams, to learning to live by your truth, your love. Respect and honor the best that is within you. And remember that all things can be medicine—a good workout, a ride in the wind, a beautiful flower, a hug, a kiss, a moment alone, shared laughter with friends, a lovely meal, an intuitive flash, a moment of acceptance, a change in awareness, a connection to the living, healing force within you.

MODIFYING THE WAY YOU EAT

FOR MOST PEOPLE TODAY it is important to recognize that convenience has become more important than nutrition, in part due to overly busy schedules and less awareness about the impact that food has on our lives. In this section we present many possible ways to move to better nutrition. The approach is to recognize harmful foods and ones most in need of being added, and to encourage changes slowly but surely.

Restaurant foods and convenience foods offer the same drawbacks:

Preservatives	many are known carcinogens
Oils	hydrogenated and partially hydrogenated oils, lard, low quality oils such as cottonseed and palm, excessive use of oils and fried foods
Salt	excessive use of
Sugar	excessive use of sugars of all types

The excessive use of these ingredients dulls the taste buds. When you cut back on them, don't be surprised to discover how tasty food can be.

Fresh fruits and vegetables are largely lacking in our diets. Fruits and vegetables are needed for their nutritional value and antioxidant actions.

You can eat more healthily regardless of your starting point by making a few simple changes.

GET NEEDED NUTRIENTS: Here are the basics.
- Fresh fruit or juice   2-3 servings/day
- Fresh vegetables   2-3 servings/day
- Protein   3 servings per day (3-6 oz. serving of meat is about right. Other sources include milk, cheese, tofu and tempeh.)

- Grains   3-5 servings of complex carbohydrate (whole
                            grains such as whole wheat, quinoa, oats, etc.)
- Take a greens drink for added nutrients and antioxidants.
- Use vitamin/mineral supplements as needed for your constitution.

GETTING STARTED
- *Become aware of what you eat* (and what your family eats, where appropriate). The best way is to keep a food log, but if that isn't your style, then at least pay attention to everything you are putting into your mouth.
- *Make a plan.* Where are you going to concentrate your efforts? Pick one of the lists of foods to be better managed—preservatives, oils, sugars or salt. For nutrients, start adding fruits and vegetables.
- *Select one target area as a starting point* and begin by making changes there. Depending on how imbalanced your current diet is, this single step can keep you busy for a while. For example, simply cutting back on sugars can take some time. Make changes step by step.
- *Keep at it and don't turn back.* Make changes at your own pace, progressing steadily, balancing your *doshas* along the way and you will be amazed at how much better, more energetic and happier you will feel!

RESTAURANT EATING: Begin making these changes to create new habits.
- Select fast food and other restaurants that have salad bars and pick dark green leaves (romaine, leaf lettuce, spinach—not iceberg lettuce).
- Select places that offer fresh vegetables with entrees.
- Become more selective with your ordering, avoiding high fat foods, etc.
- Request entrees that are baked or broiled.
- When feasible, request that entrees be cooked in olive oil or butter.
- Start cutting back on simple carbohydrates (i.e,. bread, pasta, desserts made with refined wheat flour).
  This approach automatically cuts back on oil, sugar and salt, in addition to adding more nutritional vegetables.

SNACKS

- Between meals eat fresh fruit or drink juice. If you are accustomed to soft drinks or sweet or salty snacks (cookies, candy bars, french fries, chips, etc.) cut back and substitute fruit.

CONVENIENCE FOODS

- The most important first step is to *start reading the labels.* It is not uncommon to find five or six sugar ingredients plus excessive oil, salt and preservatives on a label. Ingredients are listed in order. For example, if the first listed ingredient is sugar, sugar is the principal ingredient. If sugar is the last listed ingredient, there is less of it in the product than any other ingredient. You can cut back on sugar by simply selecting products that list it near the end of the list of ingredients. Sugar is called by many names: sugar, dextrin, dextrose, fructose, corn syrup and other syrups, glucose, galactose, lactose, cane juice, fruit juice concentrate, barley malt, sorbitol and any word followed by sugar (beet sugar, maple sugar, turbinado sugar, etc.).
- The second step is to *go on a treasure hunt* looking for more nutritious convenience foods. Check out gourmet, international and natural foods.

OTHER IDEAS

- *Involve your family or friends*: Set up a night or two per week to taste something new that you have discovered and get everyone's opinion.
- *Get into food as a hobby*: Browse around for good low-fat health oriented cookbooks. Make an adventure of discovering new spices and tastes.
- *Create quick meals*: It's possible to make nutritious quick meals that do not take more than 15 to 20 minutes to prepare. Involve family members and it can probably take even less time. All you need to do is start checking out quick meal recipe books and looking at the preparation times in standard cookbooks. You do not need to slave in the kitchen in order to serve nutritious meals.

For the most part, the changes we have suggested aren't based on total avoidance of fast food, other restaurants or convenience foods. You just have to learn to select what you eat. Bon appetit!

FOOD PLAN FOR MANAGING
VATA, PITTA AND KAPHA

THE FOLLOWING FOOD PLAN separates foods into groups that increase or decrease *vata, pitta* and *kapha*. The plan is based on the work of Dr. Vasant Lad, who has analyzed the qualities of each food, its initial and post-digestion effects, whether the food is heating or cooling, and which tastes are predominant.[1] His more detailed analysis, as well as his food combining chart, can be found in the cookbook he prepared with his wife, Usha Lad, *Ayurvedic Cooking for Self Healing*.[2] For our purposes, general categories suffice.

These food lists are prepared with all *vata, pitta* and *kapha* conditions in mind. With practice you will begin to differentiate between those foods which are most related to your particular conditions and those that are not. For example, if you have no concerns about gas or constipation, both *vata* conditions, you will not need to be as concerned about those foods which most readily increase those conditions: beans, cauliflower, brussel sprouts, broccoli and cabbage. If you have no problems with mucus but are concerned about water retention, both *kapha* conditions, you would omit foods that contain excess water from your diet but not be as concerned about dairy. If you have no problem with weight, you would not need to be as concerned about oil, carbohydrate and sugar intake.

Specific adjustments may also need to be made for individual responses to food allergens and strength of digestion. Additionally, you may find it helpful to make adjustments according to season, weather and even time of day. With seasons, *kapha* conditions increase most during the winter when congestion and colds are predominant. We also get more congested, feel heavier, and are more prone to depression during periods of coldness, cloudiness and rain. The morning period from 6:00 AM to

10:00 AM and the evening period from 6:00 PM to 10:00 PM are the times when we experience the most mucus congestion and heaviness, often needing to work quietly and move more slowly. In contrast, *pitta* conditions flare up during the hottest times, summer by season and the warmest time of day. We are more prone to become agitated, angry, critical, etc., whenever a really hot day occurs. And we are far more active from 10:00 AM to 2:00 PM, the *pitta* periods of the day. Often *pitta* symptoms of indigestion or heartburn occur from 10:00 PM to 2:00 AM. *Vata* conditions are aggravated by changes of season, especially spring and fall. Typically, winds blow more then and weather patterns shift frequently. Any weather that is shifting, especially windy weather, unsettles *vata*. For most of us, the period from 2:00 PM to 6:00 PM brings on some sense of spaciness and is not usually as productive as mid-day. During this time many reach for a stimulant and sugar. It's no accident that British Tea Time is around 4:00 PM, when many are looking for something as a "pick up."

If *vata, pitta* and *kapha* are all out of balance, there are two ways to proceed. The easiest way is to look over lists and start where food selection is easiest for your current lifestyle. The more accurate but difficult way is to take a highlighter and mark those foods which appear in the OK column for all three *doshas*. Choices will be limited, but if you have discipline try this approach. Don't grandstand and try to do everything at once.

You will notice that those foods on the recommended list for each *dosha* are in categories.

Vata Conditions: When *vata* is too high, it can be decreased by sweet, sour and salty tastes. It is increased by astringent, pungent and bitter tastes.

Pitta Conditions:. When *pitta* is too high, it can be decreased by bitter, sweet and astringent tastes. It is increased by pungent, sour and salty tastes.

Kapha Conditions: When *kapha* is too high, it can be decreased by astringent, bitter and pungent tastes. It is increased by sweet, sour and salty tastes.

Food Guidelines for Vata

Anything you eat that has the qualities of *vata* will increase *vata*. *Vata* qualities are dry, light, cold, mobile, rough and clear. The tastes that aggravate *vata* are astringent, pungent and bitter, such as found in raw vegetables and salad. Tastes which help decrease *vata* are sweet, sour and salty. In addition, *vata* is dry, so with meats, those cuts with a little more oil in them are recommended. That's why dark meat, which is oilier, is recommended over white meat when eating poultry.

Food with an asterisk (*) can be eaten with moderation, and those with two asterisks (**) can be eaten occasionally.

Foods that decrease Vata: Enjoy!

Fruits:

Most sweet fruit

Apples (cooked)	Lemons
Applesauce	Limes
Apricots	Mangoes
Avocado	Melons
Bananas	Oranges
Berries	Papaya
Cherries	Peaches
Coconut	Pineapple
Dates (fresh)	Plums
Figs (fresh)	Prunes (soaked)
Grapefruit	Raisins (soaked)
Grapes	Rhubarb
Kiwi	Strawberries

Vegetables

In general, cooked

Asparagus	Horseradish**
Beets	Leeks
Cabbage*	Mustard greens*
Carrots	Okra
Cauliflower*	Onions (cooked)*
Cilantro	Parsnip
Cucumber	Peas (cooked)
Daikon radish*	Potatoes, sweet
Fennel (Anise)	Pumpkin
Garlic	Radishes (cooked)*
Green beans	Squash, summer & winter
Green chilies	Tomatoes (cooked)**

Foods that increase Vata: Avoid!

Most dried fruit

Apples (raw)
Cranberries
Dates (dry)
Figs (dry)
Pears
Persimmons
Pomegranates
Raisins (dry)
Prunes (dry)
Watermelon

Frozen, raw or dried

Artichoke	Jerusalem
Beet greens**	artichoke*
Bitter melon	Kale
Broccoli	Kohlrabi
Brussels sprouts	Leafy greens*
Burdock root	Lettuce*
Cabbage (raw)	Mushrooms
Cauliflower (raw)	Olives, green
Celery	Onions (raw)
Corn (fresh)**	Parsley*
Dandelion greens	Peas (raw)
Eggplant	

Vata: Enjoy!

Watercress
Zucchini

Grains**

Amaranth*
Durham flour
Oats (cooked)
Pancakes
Quinoa
Rice (all kinds)
Seitan (wheat meat)
Sprouted wheat bread (Essene)
Wheat

**Always use suitable grains when "generic"
categories are listed.

Legumes

Lentils (red)
Miso**
Mung beans
Mung dal
Soy cheese*
Soy milk*
Soy sauce*
Soy sausages*
Tur dal
Urad dal

Dairy

Most dairy is good!

Butter	Ghee (clarified butter)
Buttermilk	Goat's cheese
Butter	Goat's milk
Cheese (soft)	Sour cream*
Cottage cheese	Yogurt (diluted & spiced)
Cow's milk	

Animal Foods

Beef	Salmon
Buffalo	Sardines
Chicken (dark)	Seafood
Duck	Shrimp
Eggs	Tuna
Fish (freshwater)	Turkey (dark)

Vata: Avoid!

Peppers,	Spinach (raw)*
sweet & hot	Sprouts*
Potatoes, white	Tomatoes (raw)
Radish (raw)	Turnip greens*
Spaghetti squash*	Turnips

Barley	Museli
Bread (with yeast)	Oat bran
Buckwheat	Oats (dry)
Cereals (cold,	Pasta**
dry, puffed)	Polenta**
Corn	Rice cakes**
Couscous	Rye
Crackers	Spelt
Granola	Tapioca
Millet	Wheat bran

Aduki beans	Pinto beans
Black beans	Soy beans
Black-eyed peas	Soy flour
Chick peas	Soy powder
(garbanzos)	Split peas
Kidney beans	Tempeh
Lentils (brown)	Tofu*
Lima beans	White beans
Navy beans	
Peas (dried)	

Cheese (hard)
Yogurt (plain, frozen or with fruit)

Chicken (white)*
Lamb
Pork
Rabbit
Turkey (white)
Venison

Vata: Enjoy!

Condiments

Black pepper*	Mango pickle
Chutney, mango	Mayonnaise
(sweet or spicy)	Mustard
Coriander leaves*	Pickles
DulseKelp	Salt
Ketchup	Scallions
Kombu	Seaweed
Lemon	Soy sauce
Lime	Tamari
Lime pickle	Vinegar

Nuts

In moderation:

Almonds	Macadamia nuts
Black walnuts	Peanuts**
Brazil nuts	Pecans
Cashews	Pine nuts
Coconut	Pistachios
Filberts	Walnuts
Hazelnuts	

Seeds

Chia	Pumpkin
Flax	Sesame
Halva	Sunflower
Psyllium**	Tahini

Oils

For internal & external use:
(most suitable at top of list)
Sesame
Ghee (clarified butter)
Most other oils
(Coconut and Avocado best externally only)

Beverages

Alcohol (beer or wine)*
Almond milk
Aloe vera juice
Apple cider
Apricot juice
Berry juice (except cranberry)
Carrot juice
Chai (hot spiced milk)
Cherry juice
Grain "coffee"

Vata: Avoid!

Chili peppers*
Chocolate
Horseradish
Sprouts*

None

Popcorn

Flax seed

Apple juice
Black tea
Caffeinated beverages
Carbonated drinks
Carob*
Chocolate milk
Coffee
Cold dairy drinks
Cranberry juice
Iced tea

Vata: Enjoy!

Grape juice
Grapefruit juice
Lemonade
Mango juice
Miso broth
Orange juice
Papaya juice
Peach nectar
Pineapple juice
Rice milk
Sour juices
Soy milk (hot and spiced)*

Herb Teas:

Ajwan	Kukicha*
Bancha	Lavender
Basil**	Lemon grass
Chamomile	Licorice
Cinnamon**	Marshmallow
Clove	Oat straw
Comfrey	Orange peel
Elder Flower	Peppermint
Eucalyptus	Raspberry*
Fennel	Rosehips
Fenugreek	Saffron
Ginger (fresh)	Sarasaparilla
Hawthorn	Sassafras
Juniper berry	Spearmint

Spices

All spices are good!

Ajwan	Fenugreek*
Allspice	Garlic
Almond extract	Ginger
Anise	Mace
Asafeotida (hing)	Marjoram
Basil	Mint
Bay leaf	Mustard seeds
Black pepper	Nutmeg
Cardamom	Orange peel
Cayenne*	Oregano
Cinnamon	Paprika
Cloves	Parsley
Coriander	Peppermint
Cumin	Poppyseeds
Dill	Rosemary
Fennel	Saffron

Vata: Avoid!

Icy cold drinks
Mixed vegetable juice
Pear juice
Pomegranate juice
Prune juice**
Soy milk (cold)
Tomato juice**
V-8 juice
Vegetable bouillon

Herb Teas:

Alfalfa**	Jasmine**
Barley**	Lemon balm**
Blackberry	Mormon tea
Borage**	Nettle**
Burdock	Passion flower**
Catnip*	Red clover**
Chicory*	Red Zinger**
Chrysanthemum*	Strawberry*
Corn silk	Violet*
Dandelion	Wintergreen*
Ginseng	Yarrow
Hibiscus	Yerba Mate**
Hops**	
Hyssop**	

Caraway

Vata: Enjoy!

Salt   Thyme
Savory   Turmeric
Spearmint   Vanilla
Tarragon   Wintergreen

Sweeteners

Barley malt   Molasses
Fructose   Rice syrup
Fruit juice   Stevia
  concentrates Sucanat
Honey (raw)   Turbinado

Food Supplements

Aloe vera juice*
Bee pollen
Minerals: Calcium, copper, iron
  magnesium, zinc
Royal jelly
Spiralina
Chlorella
Vitamins A, B, B12, C, D, E
Green Magic or Greens+

Vata: Avoid!

Maple syrup**
White sugar

Barley green
Brewer's yeast

Food Guidelines for Pitta

Pitta qualities include hot, sharp, light, oily, liquid, spreading (mobile) and a fleshy smell. The associated tastes, pungent, sour and salty, increase *pitta* while bitter, astringent and sweet decrease it. When selecting those foods that are most important for you to eat or avoid eating, think of the qualities you are experiencing. If you have problems with excessive acid (as with "heartburn" and acid indigestion), then start eliminating acidic foods right away (oranges, grapefruit, lemons, vinegars, pickles and anything with tomato in it). If, however, you suffer from heat related problems, such as feeling too hot, developing frequent fevers and even feeling "hotheaded," then start eliminating hot spices, especially chilies in any form.

Foods that decrease Pitta: Enjoy!

Fruits
Generally most sweet fruit

Apples (sweet)	Mangoes (ripe)
Apricots (sweet)	Melons
Avocado	Oranges (sweet)
Berries (sweet)	Pears
Cherries (sweet)	Pineapple (sweet)
Coconut	Plums (sweet)
Dates	Pomegranates
Figs	Prunes
Grapes (red & purple)	Raisins
Limes*	Watermelon

Vegetables
In general sweet & bitter

Artichoke	Okra
Asparagus	Olives, black
Beets (cooked)	Onions (cooked)
Broccoli	Parsley
Brussels sprouts	Parsnips
Cabbage	Peas
Carrots (cooked	Peppers, sweet
Cauliflower	Potatoes,
Celery	sweet & white
Cilantro	Pumpkin
Cucumber	Radishes (cooked)
Dandelion greens	Rutabaga
Fennel (Anise)	Spaghetti squash
Green beans	Spinach (cooked)**
Jerusalem artichoke	Sprouts (not spicy)
Kale	Squash,
Leafy greens	winter & summer
Leeks (cooked)	Watercress*
Lettuce	Wheat grass sprouts
Mushrooms	Zucchini

Grains**

Amaranth	Oats (cooked)
Barley	Pasta
Cereal, dry	Rice (basmati,
Couscous	white, wild)
Crackers	Rice cakes
Durham flour	Spelt
Granola	Sprouted wheat
Oat bran	bread (Essene)

Foods that increase Pitta: Avoid!

Generally most sour fruit

Apples (sour)	Mangoes (green)
Apricots (sour)	Oranges (sour)
Bananas	Papaya*
Berries (sour)	Peaches
Cherries (sour)	Persimmons
Cranberries	Pineapple (sour)
Grapefruit	Plums (sour)
Grapes (green)	Rhubarb
Kiwi**	Strawberries
Lemons	

In general pungent

Beet greens
Beets (raw)
Carrots (raw)*
Corn (fresh)**
Daikon radish
Eggplant**
Garlic
Green chilies
Horseradish
Leeks (raw)
Mustard greens
Olives, green
Onions (raw)
Peppers (hot)
Radishes (raw)
Spinach (raw)
Tomatoes
Turnip greens
Turnips

Bread (with yeast)	Rice (brown)**
Buckwheat	Rye
Corn	
Millet	
Museli**	
Oats (dry)	
Polenta**	
Quinoa	

Pitta: Enjoy!

Tapioca
Wheat
Wheat bran
**Always use suitable grains
   when "generic" foods are listed

Legumes

Aduki beans
Black beans
Chick peas (garbanzos)
Kidney beans
Lentils, brown & red
Lima beans
Mung beans
Navy beans
Peas (dried)
Pinto beans
Soy beans
Soy cheese
Soy flour*
Soy milk
Soy powder*
Split peas
Tempeh
Tofu
White beans

Dairy

Butter (unsalted)
Cheese (soft, not aged, unsalted)
Cottage cheese
Cow's milk
Ghee (clarified butter)
Goat's milk
Goat's cheese (soft, unsalted)
Ice cream
Yogurt (freshly made & diluted)

Animal Foods

Buffalo
Chicken (white)
Eggs (white only)
Fish (freshwater)
Rabbit
Shrimp*
Turkey (white)
Venison

Condiments

Black pepper*
Chutney, mango (sweet)
Coriander leaves
Lime*
Sprouts

Pitta: Avoid

Miso
Soy sauce
Soy sausages

Butter (salted)
Buttermilk
Cheese (hard)
Sour cream
Yogurt (plain, frozen or w/fruit)

Beef
Chicken (dark)
Duck
Eggs (yolk)
Fish (sea)
Lamb
Pork
Salmon
Sardines
Tuna
Turkey (dark)

Chili pepper
Chocolate
Chutney,
   mango (spicy)
Horseradish
Kelp
Ketchup
Mustard
Lemon
Lime pickle
Mango pickle
Mayonnaise

Pitta: Enjoy!

Pitta: Avoid

Pickles	Soy sauce
Salt (in excess)	Tamari*
Scallions	Vinegar
Seaweed	

Nuts

Almonds (soaked and peeled)
Coconut

Almonds (with skin)	Macadamia
Black walnuts	nuts
Brazil nuts	Peanuts
Cashews	Pecans
Filberts	Pine nuts
Hazelnuts	Pistachios
	Walnuts

Seeds

Flax
Popcorn (no salt, buttered)
Psyllium
Pumpkin*
Sunflower

Chia
Sesame
Tahini

Oils

For internal & external use:
   (most suitable at top of list)
Sunflower
Ghee (clarified butter)
Olive
Soy
Flaxseed
Evening Primrose Oil
Walnut
External only:
Avocado
Coconut

Almond
Apricot
Corn
Safflower
Sesame

Beverages

Alcohol, beer*
Aloe vera juice
Apple juice
Apricot juice
Berry juice (sweet)
Black tea
Carob
Chai (hot, spiced milk)*
Cherry juice (sweet)
Cool dairy drinks
Grain "coffee"
Grape juice

Alcohol (hard or wine)
Apple cider
Berry juice (sour)
Caffeinated beverages
Carbonated drinks
Carrot juice
Cherry juice (sour)
Chocolate milk
Coffee
Cranberry juice
Grapefruit juice
Iced tea

Pitta: Enjoy!

Mango juice
Mixed veg. juice
Peach nectar
Pear juice

Pomegranate juice
Prune juice
Rice milk
Soy milk
Vegetable bouillon

Herb teas:
Alfalfa
Bancha
Barley
Blackberry
Borage
Burdock
Catnip
Chamomile
Chicory
Chrysanthemum
Cornsilk
Dandelion
Elder flower
Fennel
Ginger (fresh)
Hibiscus
Hops
Jasmine
Lavender

Lemon balm
Lemon grass
Licorice
Marshmallow
Nettle
Oat straw
Orange peel*
Passion flower
Peppermint
Raspberry
Red clover
Saffron
Sarasparilla
Spearmint
Strawberry
Violet
Wintergreen
Yarrow

Spices
Basil (fresh)
Black pepper*
Cardamom*
Cinnamon
Coriander
Cumin
Dill
Fennel
Ginger (fresh)
Mint
Orange peel*
Parsley*
Peppermint
Saffron
Spearmint
Turmeric
Vanilla*
Wintergreen

Pitta: Avoid

Icy cold drinks
Lemonade
Orange juice*
Miso broth*

Papaya juice
Pineapple juice
Tomato juice
V-8 juice
Sour juices

Herb teas:
Basil**
Cinnamon**
Clove
Eucalyptus
Fenugreek
Ginger (dry)
Ginseng
Hawthorn
Hyssop
Juniper berry
Mormon tea
Red Zinger
Rosehip**
Sage
Sassafras
Yerba Mate

Allspice
Almond extract
Anise
Asafoetida (hing)
Basil (dry)
Bay leaf
Caraway*
Cayenne
Cloves
Fenugreek
Garlic
Ginger (dry)
Mace
Marjoram
Mustard seeds
Nutmeg
Oregano
Paprika

Poppy seeds
Rosemary
Sage
Salt
Savory
Star anise
Tarragon*
Thyme

Pitta: Enjoy!

Sweeteners

Barley malt	Rice syrup
Fructose	Stevia
Fruit juice	Sucanat
concentrates	Turbinado
Maple syrup	

Food Supplements

Aloe vera juice
Barley green
Brewer's yeast
Minerals: calcium, magnesium, zinc
Spiralina and chlorella
Vitamins D, E

Green Magic or Greens+

Pitta: Avoid

Honey*
Molasses

Amino acids
Bee pollen**
Royal jelly**
Minerals: copper, iron
Vitamins A, B, B12, C

Food Guidelines for Kapha

Kapha qualities are heavy, slow, cool, smooth, dense, oily, soft and static. It is easy to identify foods with these qualities: desserts, casseroles, sauces and anything cooked in oil. The associated tastes that increase *kapha* are sweet, salty and sour. The tastes that decrease *kapha* are astringent, bitter and pungent, such as found in salads and green vegetables. Become aware of the qualities that are excessive for you. For example, those who suffer from water retention problems have to be more careful with salty foods and foods that contain excessive water (such as melons and certain vegetables). Those who are concerned about congestion need to pay attention most closely to wheat and dairy products, both of which increase mucus. And those concerned about easy weight gain, slow metabolism and malabsorption need to pay special attention to sugar and many carbohydrates (wheat and most grains).

Foods that decrease Kapha: Enjoy!

Fruits

Generally most astringent fruit

Apples	Cherries
Applesauce	Cranberries
Apricots	Figs (dry)*
Berries	Peaches

Foods that increase Kapha: Avoid!

Generally most sweet & sour fruit

Avocado	Figs (fresh)
Bananas	Grapefruit
Coconut	Grapes*
Dates	Kiwi

Kapha: Enjoy!

Pears
Persimmons
Pomegranates
Prunes
Raisins
Strawberries*

Kapha: Avoid!

Lemons*	Pineapple
Limes*	Plums
Mangos**	Rhubarb
Melons	Watermelon
Oranges	
Papaya	

Vegetables

In general pungent & bitter

Artichoke	Leafy greens
Asparagus	Leeks
Beet greens	Lettuce
Beets	Mushrooms
Broccoli	Mustard greens
Brussels sprouts	Okra
Cabbage	Onions
Carrots	Parsley
Cauliflower	Peas
Celery	Peppers, sweet & hot
Cilantro	Potatoes, white
Corn	Radishes
Daikon radish	Rutabaga
Dandelion greens	Spinach
Eggplant	Sprouts
Fennel (Anise)	Squash (summer)
Garlic	Tomatoes (cooked)
Green beans	Turnip greens
Green chilies	Turnips
Horseradish	Watercress
Jerusalem artichoke	Wheat grass sprouts
Kale	

In general sweet & juicy

Cucumber
Olives, black or green
Parsnips**
Potatoes, sweet
Pumpkin
Spaghetti squash*
Tomatoes (raw)
Zucchini

Grains**

Amaranth*	Museli
Barley	Oat bran
Buckwheat	Oats (dry)
Cereal (cold,	Polenta
dry or puffed)	Rice (basmati, wild)*
Corn	Rye
Couscous	Sprouted wheat
Crackers	bread (Essene)
Durham flour*	Tapioca
Granola	Wheat bran
Millet	

Bread (with yeast)
Oats (cooked)
Pasta**
Quinoa*
Rice (brown, white)
Rice cakes**
Spelt*
Wheat

**Always use suitable grains when
"generic" foods are listed

Kapha: Enjoy!

Legumes

Aduki beans	Navy beans
Black beans	Peas (dried)
Black-eyed peas	Pinto beans
Chick peas	Soy milk
(garbanzos)	Soy sausages
Lentils	Split peas
(red & brown)	Tempeh
Lima beans	Tofu (hot)*
Miso	White beans

Dairy

Butter (unsalted)**
Cottage Cheese (from skimmed goat's milk)
Ghee* (clarified butter)
Goat's cheese (unsalted & not aged)*
Goat's milk (skim only)
Yogurt (diluted)

Animal Foods

Chicken (white)
Eggs
Fish (freshwater)
Rabbit
Shrimp
Turkey (white)
Venison

Condiments

Black pepper
Chili peppers
Chutney, mango (spicy)
Coriander leaves
Horseradish
Mustard (without vinegar)
Scallions
Sprouts

Nuts

Almonds (soaked & peeled)**

Kapha: Avoid!

Kidney beans
Mung beans*
Mung dal
Soy beans
Soy cheese
Soy flour
Soy powder
Soy sauce
Tofu (cold)

Butter (salted)
Buttermilk*
Cheese (soft & hard)
Cow's milk
Ice cream
Sour cream
Yogurt (plain, frozen or w/fruit)

Beef	Salmon
Buffalo	Sardines
Chicken (dark)	Tuna
Duck	Turkey (dark)
Fish (sea)	
Lamb	
Pork	

Chocolate	Mango pickle
Chutney,	Mayonnaise
mango (sweet)	Pickles
Dulse*	Salt
Kelp	Seaweed*
Ketchup	Soy sauce
Lemon*	Tamari
Lime	Vinegar
Lime pickle	

Black walnuts	Macadamia nuts
Brazil nuts	Peanuts
Cashews	Pecans
Coconut	Pine nuts
Filberts	Pistachios
Hazelnuts	Walnuts

Kapha: Enjoy!

Seeds
Chia
Flax*
Popcorn (no salt, no butter)
Psyllium**
Pumpkin*
Sunflower*

Oils
Internally & externally in small amounts:
Corn
Sunflower
Ghee (clarified butter)
Almond
Flaxseed**

Beverages
Alcohol (dry wine, red or white)
Aloe vera juice
Apple cider
Apple juice*
Apricot juice
Berry juice
Black tea (spiced)
Carob
Carrot juice
Cherry juice (sweet)
Cranberry juice
Grain "coffee"
Grape juice
Mango juice
Mixed veg. juice
Peach nectar
Pear juice
Pomegranate juice
Prune juice
Soy milk (hot & spiced)
Vegetable bouillon

Herb teas:
Alfalfa	Borage
Barley	Burdock
Basil	Catnip
Blackberry	Chamomile

Kapha: Avoid!

Sesame
Tahini

Avocado
Apricot
Coconut
Olive
Evening Primrose Oil
Safflower
Sesame
Soy
Walnut

Alcohol (beer, hard, sweet wine)
Caffeinated beverages**
Carbonated drinks
Chai (hot, spiced milk)*
Cherry juice (sour)
Chocolate milk
Coffee
Cold dairy drinks
Grapefruit juice
Iced tea
Icy cold drinks
Lemonade
Miso broth
Orange juice
Papaya juice
Pineapple juice*
Rice milk
Sour juices
Soy milk (cold)
Tomato juice
V-8 juice

Herb teas:
Comfrey
Marshmallow
Red Zinger
Rosehip**

Kapha: Enjoy!

Chicory
Chrysanthemum
Cinnamon
Clove
Corn silk
Dandelion
Elder flower
Eucalyptus
Fennel*
Fenugreek
Ginger
Ginseng*
Hibiscus
Hops
Hyssop
Jasmine
Juniper berry
Lavender
Lemon balm
Lemon grass

Licorice*
Mormon tea
Nettle
Oat straw
Orange peel
Passion flower
Peppermint
Raspberry
Red clover
Saffron
Sage
Sarsaparilla*
Sassafras
Spearmint
Strawberry
Violet
Wintergreen
Yarrow
Yerba Mate

Spices

All spices are good!

Allspice
Almond extract
Anise
Asafoetida (hing)
Basil
Bay leaf
Black pepper
Caraway
Cardamom
Cayenne
Cinnamon
Cloves
Coriander
Cumin
Dill
Fennel*
Fenugreek
Garlic
Ginger
Mace

Marjoram
Mint
Mustard seeds
Nutmeg
Orange peel
Oregano
Paprika
Parsley
Peppermint
Poppy seeds
Rosemary
Saffron
Sage
Savory
Spearmint
Star anise
Tarragon
Thyme
Turmeric
Vanilla*
Wintergreen

Kapha: Avoid!

Salt

Kapha: Enjoy!

Sweeteners
Fruit juice concentrates
Honey (raw & unprocessed)*
Stevia

*Don't cook with honey. Heat changes honey into a substance that is difficult for the body to digest.

Food Supplements
Aloe vera juice
Barley green
Bee Pollen
Brewer's yeast
Minerals: copper, calcium, iron
    magnesium, zinc
Royal jelly
Spiralina and chlorella
Vitamins A, B, B12, C, D, E
Green Magic or Greens+

Kapha: Avoid!

Barley malt	Rice syrup
Fructose	Sucanat
Maple syrup	Turbinado
Molasses	White sugar

Resources

Ayuuvedic Formulas

All Ayurvedic formulas suggested in Chapter Eight on treatment can be ordered from:

Banyan Botanicals
P.O. Box 13002
Albuquerque, NM 87192
800-953-6424
505-244-1880 / 505-244-1878 Fax

Natural Food Stores

Many of the foods and supplements suggested throughout this book are available through your local natural food store. For example:

- Multi Vitamin/Mineral Supplements
- Flaxseed Oil and Seeds
- Organically grown fruits, vegetables and meats

The packed shelves in natural food stores contain many labels, and choosing a product can be difficult. We recommend three labels that are readily available, good quality, and inexpensive—NOW, Nature's Plus, and Jarrow. If you have access to the internet, www. ConsumerLab.com is a good resource. This independent laboratory offers quality comparison of many lablels.

Greens Drinks

If you can't find a greens drink in your local store, Greens+ and Green Magic can be ordered from the following sources:

Greens+ is available from:
Orange Peel Enterprises, Inc.
2183 Ponce de Leon Circle
Vero Beach, FL 32960
1-800-643-1210
www.greensplus.com

Green Magic is available from:
New Spirit Naturals
458 West Arrow
San Dimas, CA 91773
909-592-4445
1-800-922-2766 (outside California)

Real Salt

Real Salt, the form of rock salt we recommend, is available in some natural food stores or from the following source:
Redmond Minerals
P.O. Box 219
Redmond, UT 84652
800-367-7258
www.realsalt.com

Sea Salt

A number of unrefined sea salts are available in your local store. A high quality Celtic sea salt can be ordered from:
The Grain and Salt Society
P.O. Box DD
Magalia, CA 95954
916-872-5800

Herbamare and Trocomare

If you can't find these recommended herbal salts, try ordering from:
Bioforce of America, Ltd.
P.O. Box 507
Kinderhook, NY 12106
800-445-8802

Sea Vegetables

Delicious and convenient shakers of sea vegetables sold under the label of Sea Seasonings from Maine Coast Sea Vegetables are available in many natural food stores. Try Kelp Granules, Dulse Granules or, if you prefer a bit more taste, select Kelp Granules with Cayenne or Dulse Granules with Ginger. If you can't find these products, contact:
Maine Coast Sea Vegetables
Franklin, ME 04634
207-565-2907
www.seaveg.com

For high quality bulk sea vegetables for medicinal and culinary use, contact:
Maine Seaweed Company
PO Box 57
Steuben, ME 04680
207-546-2003

Charts and Mirrors for Reading the Iris
Natural Books & Products
1718 East Valley Pkwy.
Suite C
Escondido, CA 92027
619-743-1790

Labs for Functional Assessment
Great Smokies Diagnostic Laboratory
63 Zillicoa Street
Ashville, NC 28801
800-522-4762
Fax: 562-592-3383

We recommend Great Smokies Diagnostic Laboratory, because that is the one we use. However, there are a number of other good labs that specialize in functional assessment.

The Authors: To contact either of the authors

Dr. Margaret Smith Peet   Dr. Shoshana Zimmerman
mspeet@aol.com   drshoshana@drshoshana.com
                                             www.drshoshana.com

Dr. Peet and Dr. Zimmerman are available for private consultations via phone or e-mail.

NOTES

Chapter 1

[1] Much of this material was formulated in western terms by Michael Dick, a classical Ayurvedic scholar associated with the Ayurvedic Institute in Albuquerque, NM. Michael Dick has the ability to analyze and apply ancient concepts from a fresh point of view that keeps Ayurveda dynamic.

[2] We all have a level of awareness or consciousness regardless of how we define spirit. The word spirit can conjure up images of non-human entities, such as ghosts or angels, or have religious connotations. Consciousness or awareness, on the other hand, implies understanding. The greater one's awareness, the greater one's understanding. Differences in levels of understanding are sometimes referred to as lower or higher states of consciousness, and these levels in turn affect how we interpret the world.

[3] We use these Sanskrit words because there are no English words to fully describe these concepts. Throughout this book we will use Sanskrit or Chinese terms only when there are no adequate English words.

[4] Lad, Vasant. *The Complete Book of Ayurvedic Home Remedies*. New York: Harmony Books, 1998, p. 42.

Chapter 2

[1] Kushi, Michio. *Your Face Never Lies*. Wayne, NJ: Avery Publishing Group, p. 11.

[2] Much of the material on face analysis can be found in the work of Dr. Vasant Lad, an Ayurvedic physician, and Wataru Ohashi, a Shiatsu master. The material is not exclusive to them. Rather, they have made available to us in the West information that has been part of their traditions for thousands of years. Dr. Peet has been a student of both of these men. Dr. Zimmerman has been a student of Dr. Lad and has studied Ohashi's writings. We do not attempt to carefully document each marking and its interpretation, as if we must credit every thought to Dr. Lad or Ohashi. After years of being immersed in these systems we wish to credit both men for sharing knowledge from their traditions with us, and we will do our best to present it in terms that we Westerners can readily understand. Our gratefulness to these teachers cannot be expressed in words but is deeply felt in the heart. For those who would like to read the works of either, we refer you to the following books

that are also listed in the bibliography: Dr. Vasant Lad. *Ayurveda: The Science of Self-Healing*; *The Complete Book of Ayurvedic Home Remedies*; *Ayurvedic Cooking for Self-Healing*; *The Yoga of Herbs*; *Secrets of the Pulse*. Volume I of a proposed three volume textbook on Ayurveda will be published in 2001. Wataru Ohashi, *Reading the Body: Ohashi's Book of Oriental Diagnosis*.

[3] Ohashi, Wataru and Tom Monte. *Reading the Body: Ohashi's Book of Oriental Diagnosis*. New York: Penguin/Arkana, 1991, pp. 37-39.

[4] Marieb, Elaine N. *Human Anatomy and Physiology*. Redwood City, CA: Benjamin/Cummings Publishing Co., 1989, p. 879.

[5] Marieb, pp. 668-669.

[6] Ohashi, p. 57.

[7] Ohashi, p. 57.

[8] Ohashi, p. 60.

[9] Ohashi, p. 59.

[10] Ohashi, p 59.

[11] Ohashi, pp. 65-66.

Chapter 3

[1] Marieb, p. 762.

[2] Ohashi, p. 73.

[3] Kaptchuk, Ted J., OMD. *The Web That Has No Weaver: Understanding Chinese Medicine*. New York: Congdon & Weed, 1983, p. 147.

[4] Maciocia, Giovanni. *Tongue Diagnosis in Chinese Medicine*. Seattle: Eastland Press, 1987, p. 16.

[5] Maciocia, p. 16.

[6] Kaptchuk, pp. 147-148.

[7] Maciocia, p. 38.

[8] Maciocia, p. 59.

[9] Maciocia, p. 67.

[10] Ohashi, p. 72.

[11] Kaptchuk, p. 148.

[12] Ohashi, pp. 72-73.

[13] Ohashi, p. 73.

[14] Lad, Dr. Vasant. *Ayurveda: The Science of Self-Healing*. Wilmot, WI: Lotus Light, 1984, p. 60.

[15] Many labs do not test for RT3 and therefore give an incorrect figure for the T3 reading. If you have a thyroid problem, be sure that RT3 is included in the test results.

Chapter 4

[1] We wish to thank Hart de Fouw for his workshops on hand analysis. Much of this material is based on Ayurvedic teachings that he has brought to the West. In addition, we have drawn on the expertise of Andrew Fitzherbert in his book *Hand Psychology*, Garden City Park, NY: Avery Publishing, 1989. We are grateful for having obtained the classic book on hand analysis by Mrs. Robinson, *The Graven Palm: A Manual of the Science of Palmistry*, London: Edward Arnold, 1911 (out of print). The traditions of the East and West are amazingly compatible.

[2] Our thanks to Hart de Fouw for his help in the preparation of these markings.

[3] Dr. Vasant Lad. *Ayurveda: The Science of Self-Healing*, p. 66.

Chapter 5

[1] There are a variety of charts that show these areas. For a detailed chart we recommend Bernard Jensen's *Chart to Iridology* because it is easy to use. Harry Wolfe has developed a slightly different chart but it is, in our opinion, difficult to use. Dr. Vasant Lad has a simple chart showing body organs on the iris but it is not published.

[2] Most of our information came through Ayurvedic teachings and extensive coursework with Dr. Harry Wolfe and Dr. Ellen Tart, who introduced us to both Bernard Jensen's and Harry Wolfe's systems as well as to other systems.

[3] Harry Wolfe lecture 9/24/95 and work of Glenda Schneider in *Iris Analysis*.

[4] We are especially appreciative of Dr. Ellen Tart's efforts to teach us iridology. Most of the information in this section comes from attending her workshops during 1995 and 1996.

[5] Kushi, pp. 35-36.

[6] Ohashi, pp. 76-77; Kushi, p. 35.

[7] Ohashi, p. 153.

[8] Ohashi, pp. 154-156.

[9] Ohashi, p. 155.

[10] Ohashi, p. 155.

Chapter 6

[1] Chinese medicine also uses the radial pulse in diagnosis. However, the Chinese system, including the position of the fingers, is somewhat different from that of Ayurveda. In the Chinese system, the index finger is placed on the side of this bone next to the hand. In Ayurveda, the index finger is placed on the side of this bone away from the hand.

[2] Ayurveda also includes the concept of energy pathways, but the system is much more subtle and difficult to understand. For our purposes we will use the Chinese and Japanese concept of meridians to explain the pathways of the life force, the *chi*, because this concept is more widespread in the West and is easily understood.

[3] There are some differences in Japanese and Chinese meridian charts. We use charts based on Ohashi's Japanese system.

[4] Much of the material for this section is based on Ohashi's work.

[5] Ohashi, pp. 105-106.

[6] Ohashi, p. 107.

[7] Here in the West various writers have explained these centers well, including such people as Caroline Myss in her book *Anatomy of the Spirit* and Christiane Northrup in *Women's Bodies, Women's Wisdom*. Different authors give different names and meanings to the *chakras,* which can create some confusion.

[8] Caroline Myss, PhD. *Anatomy of the Spirit* (NY: Three Rivers Press, 1996).

Chapter 7

[1] DesMaisons, Kathleen, Ph.D. *Potatoes Not Prozac*. New York: Simon & Schuster/Fireside Books, 1998, p. 43.

[2] DesMaisons, op. cit.

[3] D'Adamo, Dr. Peter J. *Eat Right 4 Your Type*. New York: Putnam, 1996, pp. 21-23.

[4] D'Adamo, p. 23.

[5] Information from a conversation with Dr. Vasant Lad.

[6] We found an approximate 70-75% correlation comparing the items individually.

Chapter 9

[1] Walford, Roy L., MD. *The 120 Year Diet: How to Double Your Vital Years*. New York: Simon & Schuster, 1986.

[2] Stevia is an herb that we recommend in place of artificial sweeteners. Later in this chapter Stevia will be discussed in detail.

[3] Carper, Jean. *The Food Pharmacy: Dramatic New Evidence that Food Is Your Best Medicine*. New York: Bantam Books, 1988, p. 220.

[4] Carper, p. 153.

[5] Carper, p. 154. For more information about how to use cabbage juice in treatment of ulcers, see "Dr. Cheney's Antiulcer Cabbage Cocktail" on pp. 154-155.

[6] Carper, pp. 156-157.

[7] Carper, pp. 114-117.

[8] Carper, pp. 122-125.

[9] Lad, Usha & Dr. Vasant Lad. *Ayurvedic Cooking for Self-Healing*. Albuquerque: Ayurvedic Press, Second Edition, 1997, p. 184.

[10] For variations on this recipe, see *Ayurvedic Cooking for Self-Healing*.

[11] Willard, Terry, Lecture "Are Medicinal Mushrooms Magic?" Southwest Conference on Botanical Medicine, Tempe, AZ, April 10-11, 1999.

[12] For in-depth information about medicinal mushrooms, see Christopher Hobbs' book *Medicinal Mushrooms: An Exploration of Tradition, Healing & Culture*. Santa Cruz, CA: Botanica Press, 1986.

[13] Pitchford, Paul, *Healing with Whole Foods: Oriental Traditions and Modern Nutrition*. Berkeley, CA: North Atlantic Books, 1993, p. 540.

[14] Colbin, Annemarie. *Food and Healing*. New York: Ballantine Books, 1986, pp. 180-181.

[15] Kesten, Deborah. *Feeding the Body, Nourishing the Soul*. Berkeley: Conari Press, 1997, p. 3.

[16] Kesten, p. 150.

[17] Lad, Vasant. *Textbook on Ayurveda: Volume I, The History and Philosophy of Ayurveda*. Albuquerque, NM: Ayurvedic Press, to be published in 2001.

[18] Burrell's Transcripts, "Resolutions That Matter," *Oprah: The Oprah Winfrey Show*, aired January 16, 1997 (Harpo Productions, Inc., 1997), 17.

Chapter 10

[1] Cabrera, Chanchal. "Holistic herbal strategies for enhanced immune function," lecture given at the 4th International Herb Symposium, "Modern & Traditional Uses of Herbal Medicine," Wheaton College, Norton, MA, June 26-28, 1998.

[2] "Antibiotic Misuse Turns Treatable to Incurable," *New York Science Times*, Tuesday, June 13, 2000, p. F2.

[3] "Pesticides may cause brain damage in kids, study finds," *Arizona Republic*, March 18, 1999.

[4] "Threat to public health?" *Arizona Republic*, February 26, 1999, A26.

[5] "European Union proposes new steps to stop 'mad cow' disease," *San Jose Mercury News*, Thursday, November 30, 2000, p. 8A.

[6] Petersen, Melody, "Farmers' right to sue grows, raising debate on food safety," *New York Times*, June 1, 1999, A1.

[7] "Food scare is leaving tables bare in Belgium," *New York Times*, June 6, 1999, p. 15.

[8] Arnesen, E., Forde, O.H., and Thelle, D.S., "Coffee and serum cholesterol, " *British Medical Journal*, 1984, 288, p. 1,960.

[9] Boyle, C.A., Berkowitz, G.S., LiVolsi, V.A., et al., "Caffeine consumption and fibrocystic breast disease: A case control epidemiologic study," J.N.C.I., 1984, 72, pp. 1,015-19.

[10] Lang, T., Degoulet, P., Aime, F., et al., "Relationship between coffee drinking and blood pressure: Analysis of 6,321 subjects in the Paris region," *American Journal of Cardiology*, 1983, 52, pp. 1,238-42.

[11] Formann, S., Hashell, W., Vranizan, K., et al., "The association of blood pressure and dietary alcohol: Difference by age, sex and estrogen use," *American Journal of Epidemiology*, 1983, 118, pp. 497-507.

[12] Pizzorno, J.E., and Murray, M.T., *A Textbook of Natural Medicine*, John Bastyr College Publications, Seattle, WA, 1985.

[13] Murray, Michael, ND, and Joseph Pizzorno, ND. *Encyclopedia of Natural Medicine*. Rocklin, CA: Prima Publishing, 1991, p. 169.

[14] Murray and Pizzorno, p. 394.

[15] Hanington, E., "The platelet and migraine," *Headache*, 1986, 26, pp. 411-15.

[16] Murray and Pizzorno, p. 489.

[17] Ballentine, Rudolph, MD. *Radical Healing: Integrating the World's Great Therapeutic Traditions to Create a New Transformative Medicine*. New York: Harmony Books, 1999, p. 237.

[18] Cabrera, lecture.

[19] Gittleman, Ann Louise, MS, CNS. *Get the Sugar Out*. New York: Three Rivers Press, 1996, p xii.

[20] Cabrera, lecture.

[21] Gittleman, Sugar, p 12.

[22] Russell Blaylock, MD. *Excitotoxins: The Taste That Kills* (Health Press, 1994. 1-800-643-2665). Dr. H. J. Roberts, a diabetic specialist and expert on aspartame poisoning, has also written a book entitled *Defense Against Alzheimer's Disease* (1-800-814-9800).

[23] For more information about the dangers of aspartame, send a self-addressed, stamped envelope and a $1.00 donation to: Aspartame Consumer Safety Network, PO Box 780634, Dallas, TX 75378.

[24] Richard, David. *Stevia Rebaudiana: Nature's Sweet Secret*. Bloomingdale, IL, Blue Heron Press, 1996, pp. 25-26.

[25] Gittleman, Ann Louise. *Get the Salt Out*. New York: Three Rivers Press, 1996, p. 9.

[26] Gittleman, Salt, p. 15.

[27] Gittleman, Salt, p. 15.

[28] Gittleman, Salt, p. 18.

[29] Gittleman, Salt, p. 20.

[30] Gittleman, Salt, p. 33.

[31] As Russell L. Blaylock, MD, says in his book *Excitoxins: The Taste That Kills* (Health Press, 1994), "The distribution of cellular damage caused by large concentration of MSG is very similar to that seen in human cases of Alzheimer's disease."

[32] Gittleman, Salt, p. 101.

[33] Gittleman, Salt, p. 54. For more extensive information about salt, as well as excellent recipe suggestions, see *Get the Salt Out*.

[34] Weil, Andrew, "Good fats, bad fats," *Dr. Andrew Weil's Self Healing*, December 1998, p. 1.

[35] Weil, p. 1.

[36] Brody, Jane, "New look at dieting: Fat can be a friend," *New York Times Science Times*, May 25, 1999, D1.

[37] Bang, H. O. and John Dyerberg, a 1978 study published in *Lancet*, the highly respected British medical journal.

[38] Weil, p. 6.

[39] Gittleman, Ann Louise, *Beyond Pritikin*. New York: Bantam Books, 1988, p. 28.

[40] Murray, Michael T., ND. *Encyclopedia of Nutritional Supplements*. Rocklin, CA: Prima Publishing, 1996, pp. 243-244.

[41] Gittleman, *Beyond Pritikin*, p. 28.

[42] According to leading cardiac specialist and researcher, Dr. Kurt A. Oster, Chief of Cardiology Emeritus at Park City Hospital, Bridgeport, Connecticut.

[43] Gittleman, *Beyond Pritikin*, p. 32.

[44] Murray, p. 250.

Chapter 11

[1] Cabrera, lecture.

[2] Cabrera, lecture.

[3] Cabrera, lecture.

[4] F. Batmanghelidj, MD. *Your Body's Many Cries for Water*. Falls Church, VA: Global Health Solutions, 1995.

[5] Batmanghelidj, p. 6.

[6] Ropp, Thomas, "Sunday special report: Water," *The Arizona Republic*, May 30, 1999, A1.

[7] Ibid.

[8] "Drinking a lot of liquid may deter a cancer," *The New York Times*, May 6, 1999, A25.

[9] Batmanghelidj, p. 17.

[10] Batmanghelidj, p. 18.

[11] "Food-guide pyramid revised for seniors over 70," *New York Times, Science Times*, March 2, 1999.

[12] Batmanghelidj, p. 18.

[13] "Poisonous Plastics?" *Time*, March 1, 1999, p. 53.

[14] Ibid.

[15] Cabrera, lecture.

[16] "T'ai chi vs. aerobics study results surprising," *The Arizona Republic*, March 15, 1999. Report on a new study in the *Journal of the American Geriatrics Society*.

[17] Pert, Candace B., Ph.D. *Molecules of Emotion: The Science Behind Mind-Body Medicine*. New York: Touchstone, 1999.

[18] Cabrera, lecture.

[19] "S. Calif. Kids focus of pollution study," *Arizona Republic*, March 18, 1999.

Chapter 12

[1] See pages 187 - 216 of *Ayurvedic Cooking for Self-Healing* for more medicinal uses of fruits, vegetables and herbs.

[2] Pitchford, p. 505.

[3] See recipes in *Ayurvedic Cooking for Self-Healing*.

[4] Jarvis, Dr. D. C. *Vermont Folk Medicine*. New York: Crest, Fawcett World, 1969.

[5] Frawley, Dr. David and Dr. Vasant Lad. *The Yoga of Herbs*. Twin Lakes, WI: Lotus Press, 1986, p. 122.

[6] Winston, David. Lecture, "Crataegus, Cactus and Convalaria," Southwest Conference on Botanical Medicine, Tempe, AZ, April 10-11, 1999.

[7] Brody, Jane E., "Americans Gamble on Herbs as Medicine," *The New York Time Science Times*, Tuesday, February 9, 1999, p. D1.

[8]"Herbal healing," *Time*, November 23, 1998, p. 58.

[9] Frawley and Lad. *The Yoga of Herbs*, p. 123.

[10] Frawley and Lad, pp. 160-161.

[11] Simopoulos, Artemis P., M.D. and Jo Robinson. *The Omega Plan*. New York: HarperCollins, 1998, p. 149.

[12] Frawley and Lad, p. 119.

Chapter 13

[1] Material for this travel section came from the following sources:

Conversation with JaneAbrams, Clinical Herbalist, July 3, 1999.

Cascade Anderson Geller, "A Traveler's Mini-Guide, Including Natural and Conventional Remedies for Some Conditions Encountered Around the World," March 1978, Revised 1996.

Rob McCaleb, HRF President, "The Herbally Aware Traveler," from the website of the Herb Research Foundation.

Dana Myatt, ND, Lecture, "Urgent Care Herbalist," Southwest Conference on Botanical Medicine, Tempe, AZ, April 10-11, 1999.

[2] For more information about castor oil packs, see Dr. Harold J. Reilly's book, *The Edgar Cayce Handbook for Health Through Drugless Therapy*. New York: Macmillan, 1975.

Chapter 14

[1] "Information, Please: It turns out that the biological world is chock-full of it," *New York Times Book Review*, May 23, 1999, p 26.

[2] Pert, Candace B., PhD. *Molecules of Emotion: The Science Behind Mind-Body Medicine*. New York: Simon & Schuster/Touchstone, 1997, pp 286-295.

[3] Dossey, Larry, MD. *Reinventing Medicine: Beyond Mind-Body to a New Era of Healing*. San Francisco: Harper, 1999, pp. 45-59.

[4] Dossey, pp. 138-151.

[5] Lecture, "Energy Medicine in Clinical Practice," presented by Carolyn McMakin, DC, at The Seventh International Symposium on Functional Medicine, May 25, 2000 in Scottsdale, AZ.

[6] Gordon, Richard, *Quantum-Touch: The Power to Heal.* Berkeley: North Atlantic Books, 1999.

[7] Gordon, pp. 16-23.

[8] Ornish, Dean, MD. *Love & Survival: The Scientific Basis for the Healing Power of Intimacy.* New York: HarperCollins, 1998.

[9] Northrup, Christiane, MD. *Women's Bodies, Women's Wisdom: Creating Physical and Emotional Health and Healing.* New York: Bantam, 1998.

[10] Northrup, pp. 579-641.

[11] Myss, Caroline, PhD. *Anatomy of the Spirit: The Seven Stages of Power and Healing.* New York Random House, 1997.

[12] Pert, p. 245.

[13] Moyers, Bill D. *Healing and the Mind*, New York: Doubleday, 1993.

Appendix B

[1] Lad, Dr. Vasant. "Food Guideline for Basic Constitutional Types," The Ayurvedic Institute, Albuquerque, NM, 1994.

[2] Lad, Usha & Dr. Vasant Lad. *Ayurvedic Cooking for Self-Healing* (Second Edition). Albuquerque: The Ayurvedic Press, 1997.

BIBLIOGRAPHY

Balch, James F., MD and Phyllis A. Balch, CNC. *Prescription for Nutritional Healing* (Second Edition). Garden City Park, NY: Avery Publishing Group, 1997.
  The Balches have put together a useful book as a guide for alternative healing options.

Batmanghelidj, F., MD. *Your Body's Many Cries for Water: You Are Not Sick, You Are Thirsty!* (Second Edition). Falls Church, VA: Global Health Solutions, Inc., 1995.
  Although Dr. Batmanghelidj pushes his point a bit too far, there is merit in his position about the importance of water and the devastating effects of dehydration. Indeed, water is often the best medicine.

Blaylock, Russell L., MD. *Excitotoxins: The Taste That Kills*. Santa Fe: Health Press, 1997.
  An informative book about the dangers of aspartame and MSG.

Chopra, Deepak, MD. *Ageless Body, Timeless Mind: The Quantum Alternative to Growing Old*. New York: Harmony Books, 1993.
  Dr. Chopra deserves much credit for popularizing Ayurveda in the West. Through his books and lectures, he has presented many of the basic concepts and treatment approaches used by Ayurveda.

_____ *Quantum Healing: Exploring the Frontiers of Mind/Body Medicine*. New York: Bantam, 1989.

_____ *Perfect Health: The Complete Mind/Body Guide*. New York: Harmony Books, 1991.

Crawford, Amanda McQuade. *The Herbal Menopause Book: Herbs, Nutrition & Other Natural Therapies*. Freedom, CA: The Crossing Press, 1996.
  These two books are excellent resource books for choosing western herbs for women's issues. Readable and highly recommended.

_____ *Herbal Remedies for Women*. Rocklin, CA: Prima Publishing, 1997.

D'Adamo, Dr. Peter J. *Eat Right 4 Your Type: The Individualized Diet Solution to Staying Healthy, Living Longer & Achieving Your Ideal Weight*. New York: Putnam, 1996.

The approach Dr. D'Adamo develops parallels Ayurveda in the relationship of *dosha* to blood type. The dietary recommendations for each blood type also have much in common with Ayurveda.

DesMaisons, Kathleen, PhD. *Potatoes not Prozac*. New York: Simon & Schuster/ Fireside, 1998.

This book offers a clear explanation of the relationship between sugar sensitivity, insulin resistance, excessive carbohydrate intake and the development of a wide variety of common symptoms. DesMaisons offers dietary recommendations that are compatible with Ayurveda and are highly workable.

Dougans, Inge, *The Complete Illustrated Guide to Reflexology*. New York: Barnes & Noble, 1996.

This beautifully illustrated book explains the key reflex points in the feet and how they are linked to the meridians and to your major organs. Techniques for gently massaging your feet to help improve energy flow are well illustrated.

_____*The Art of Reflexology: A Step-by-Step Guide*. New York: Barnes & Noble, 1995.

Another useful book on reflexology by the same author.

Erasmus, Udo. *Fats That Heal, Fats That Kill: The Complete Guide to Fats, Oils, Cholesterol and Human Health* (Second Edition). Burnaby BC Canada: Alive Books, 1993.

Erasmus is perhaps the best authority on fats and the effects of different kinds of fats on health. This book is detailed and packed with information. Not an easy read but highly recommended.

Fitzherbert, Andrew. *Hand Psychology: A New Insight into Solving Your Problems*. Garden City Park, NY: Avery Publishing Group, 1989.

Andrew Fitzherbert's work in discussing and illustrating major hand shapes and lines is excellent. The drawings are well prepared and his explanations are clear.

Frawley, Dr. David and Dr. Vasant Lad. *The Yoga of Herbs*. Twin Lakes, WI: Lotus Press, 1992.

This book offers additional reading about herbs and their qualities from an Ayurvedic point of view. Both western and Ayurvedic herbs are included.

Gittleman, Ann Louise, MS, CNS. *Get the Salt Out: 501 Simple Ways to Cut the Salt Out of Any Diet*. New York: Three Rivers Press, 1996.

Gittleman's writing is simple, direct and informative. Her books on sugar, salt and fat give excellent insights into the health effects of these substances. Highly recommended.

_____ *Get the Sugar Out*. New York: Three Rivers Press, 1996.

_____ *Beyond Pritikin*. New York: Bantam Books, 1988.

Harman, Willis. *Global Mind Change: The Promise of the 21st Century* (Second Edition). San Francisco: Berrett-Koehler Publishers, Inc., 1998.

We agree with Willis Harman that a major global mind shift is occurring in how we view the world, a shift as major as any in history and one which will alter the way we view our bodies and our responsibility for caring for ourselves. This is a thought provoking book, particularly if you are interested in the way consciousness affects societal and even global change.

Hendler, Sheldon Saul, MD, PhD. *The Doctors' Vitamin and Mineral Encyclopedia*. New York: Simon & Schuster/Fireside, 1990.

This book is an introduction to vitamins and herbs. Dr. Hendler identifies popular claims and the scientific data to support or discredit the claims. Much research has been done since 1990, so an updated version would be useful.

Hobbs, Christopher, LAc. *Medicinal Mushrooms: An Exploration of Tradition, Healing & Culture*. Santa Cruz, CA: Botanica Press, 1986.

An informative guide to medicinal mushrooms.

Jensen, Dr. Bernard, and Dr. Donald V. Boden. *Visions of Health: Understanding Iridology*. Garden City Park, NY: Avery Publishing Group, 1992.

This little volume on iridology is an excellent and readable introduction. Highly recommended.

Kesten, Deborah. *Feeding the Body, Nourishing the Soul: Essentials of Eating for Physical, Emotional and Spiritual Well-Being*. Berkeley, CA: Conari Press, 1997.

The importance of food for the well-being of body-mind-spirit is beautifully dealt with in this book.

Kushi, Michio. *Your Face Never Lies: What Your Face Reveals About Your Health*. Wayne, NJ: Avery Publishing Group, Inc., 1983.

This thin volume is packed with information about facial markings. It can easily lead you to wanting to know more about what your face reveals.

Lad, Dr. Vasant. *Ayurveda: The Science of Self-Healing*. Wilmot, WI: Lotus Press, 1984.

This first book by Dr. Lad, published in 1984, was a pioneer work in introducing Ayurveda to readers in this country. The writing is dense and packed with information. It is considered a classic and is highly recommended. However, it is not a beginner's book. Read Morrison first and then the two books by Svoboda before attempting this book.

_____ *The Complete Book of Ayurvedic Home Remedies*. New York: Harmony Books, 1998.

Traditional Ayurvedic formulas and treatments for many different conditions are presented in this book. Also included are sections on basic Ayurvedic concepts.

_____ *Secrets of the Pulse: The Ancient Art of Ayurvedic Pulse Diagnosis*. Albuquerque: The Ayurvedic Press, 1996.

Dr. Lad's approach to pulse diagnosis is thoroughly covered in this book.

Lad, Usha and Dr. Vasant. *Ayurvedic Cooking for Self-Healing* (Second Edition). Albuquerque: The Ayurvedic Press, 1997.

This book, written for Western use, explains the Ayurvedic concept of nutrition and suggests many recipes for balancing your *doshas*. The book is particularly helpful in learning how to cook Ayurvedically. Included is an excellent section on the principles of food combining to enhance digestion.

Lininger, Skye, DC, Jonathan Wright, MD, Steve Austin, ND, Donald Brown, ND, Alan Gaby, MD. *The Natural Pharmacy*. Rocklin, CA: Prima Health, 1998.

These authors provide an abundance of information on integrative approaches to common problems. They are not trained in Ayurveda, but they are well informed about natural approaches to treating illness.

Maciocia, Giovanni. *Tongue Diagnosis in Chinese Medicine*. Seattle: Eastland Press, 1987.

This is a technical book about tongue diagnosis with some excellent photos of bodily conditions reflected on the tongue. It's a must for anyone interested in a serious study of tongue diagnosis.

Morrison, Judith H. *The Book of Ayurveda: A Holistic Approach to Health and Longevity*. New York: Simon & Schuster/Fireside, 1995.

This book on Ayurveda is an excellent introduction to the basic concepts and is a recommended companion volume to *My Doctor Says I'm Fine . . . So Why Do I Feel So Bad?* Readable and beautifully illustrated.

Murray, Michael, T., ND. *Encyclopedia of Nutritional Supplements: The Essential Guide for Improving Your Health Naturally*. Rocklin, CA: Prima Publishing, 1996.

Dr. Murray is one of the foremost leaders in the use of nutritional supplements and herbs from a western perspective.

Murray, Michael, ND, and Joseph Pizzorno, ND. *Encyclopedia of Natural Medicine* (Revised Second Edition). Rocklin, CA: Prima Publishing, 1998.

This volume is a companion to the one above.

Myss, Caroline, PhD. *Anatomy of the Spirit: The Seven Stages of Power and Healing*. New York: Three Rivers Press, 1996.

It is difficult to say too much about the pioneering work of Caroline Myss. She offers a fresh, comprehensive approach to a study of the body's energy centers as viewed from ancient mystical and religious perspectives. One of the things we like best is that she shares her extrordinary extrasensory perceptions without any apologies and presents ways of using these perceptions in a complementary way with allopathic medicine.

_____ *Why People Don't Heal and How They Can*. New York: Harmony Books, 1997.

Caroline Myss, while perhaps never a student of Ayurveda, has presented concepts of healing that parallel those of ancient Ayurveda. We applaud her work.

Northrup, Christiane, MD. *Women's Bodies, Women's Wisdom: Creating Physical and Emotional Health and Healing* (Second Edition). New York: Bantam Books, 1998.

Dr. Christiane Northrup has had a major impact on the very definition of medicine, expanding far beyond the narrow mechanistic and specialized approach of allopathic medicine to include comprehensive views of the body-mind-spirit relationship. She may never have studied Ayurveda, but the concepts she presents are quite compatible.

Ohashi, Wataru, with Tom Monte. *Reading the Body: Ohashi's Book of Oriental Diagnosis*. New York: Penguin/Arkana, 1991.

After studying Ohashi's book, you will never again view the human body in a matter of fact way. Indeed, who we are is reflected in everything about us.

Pitchford, Paul. *Healing with Whole Foods: Oriental Traditions and Modern Nutrition*. Berkeley, CA: North Atlantic Books, 1993.

This thick paperback is packed with excellent information about every food group and has general guidelines about nutition and lifestyle. The sections on fats and salt are particularly useful. Also included is a lengthy section on seaweeds, their value in the diet and even recipes for using them. Pitchford has done a beautiful job in putting together a useful book. Highly recommended.

Reilly, Dr. Harold J. *The Edgar Cayce Handbook for Health Through Drugless Therapy*. New York: Jove/HBJ, 1977.

The approach to healing outlined by Edgar Cayce has many parallels in Ayurveda. Dr. Reilly's book discusses Cayce's approach and the various herbs and substances he used, including castor oil packs.

Sharma, Hari, MD. *Freedom from Disease: How to Control Free Radicals, A Major Cause of Aging and Disease*. Toronto: Veda Publishing, 1993.

Dr. Sharma presents valuable information about the role of free radicals in the development of disease.

Simopoulos, Artemis P., MD, and Jo Robinson. *The Omega Plan: The Medically Proven Diet That Gives You the Essential Nutrients You Need*. New York: HarperCollins, 1998.

Although we do not recommend everything presented in this book, the basic guidelines are excellent. This book is a much easier read than the book on fats by Erasmus.

Smith, Trevor, MD. *Homeopathic Medicine: A Doctor's Guide to Remedies for Common Ailments*. Rochester, VT: Healing Arts Press, 1989.

As an introductory volume this book presents a multitude of remedies for common conditions in a straightforward and organized manner.

Svoboda, Dr. Robert E. *Ayurveda: Life, Health & Longevity*. New York: Penguin Books, 1992.

_____ *Prakruti: Your Ayurvedic Constitution*. Albuquerque: GEOCOM, 1989.

These two books by Dr. Svoboda are well written and present Ayurvedic concepts in understandable language. Although more advanced than the book by Judith Morrison, we recommend these books as companions to *My Doctor Says I'm Fine*.

Tierra, Michael, CA, ND, OMD. *Planetary Herbology: An Integration of Western Herbs into the Traditional Chinese and Ayurvedic Systems*. Santa Fe: Lotus Press, 1988.
> Michael Tierra's approach to herbology is similar to ours, incorporating the best of both western and eastern herbs.

Tiwari, Maya. *A Life of Balance*. Rochester, VT: Healing Arts Press, 1995.
> When Maya Tiwari, a Hindu woman who was a successful New York fashion designer, was diagnosed with terminal cancer and given little chance of survival, she claimed her roots as a Brahmin and redefined her life as a holistic being, incorporating body, mind and spirit. In this large paperback book, Tiwari describes her journey back to health and defines the importance of nutrition in relationship to constitution in living a life of balance.

Weil, Andrew, MD. *Spontaneous Healing: How to Discover and Enhance Your Body's Natural Ability to Maintain and Heal Itself*. New York: Fawcett Columbine, 1995.
> The books written by Dr. Weil have helped enormously in raising consciousness around the importance of a holistic approach to health care.

West, Peter. *The Complete Illustrated Guide to Palmistry*. New York: Barnes & Noble, 1998.
> This book presents basic concepts of hand analysis, including some helpful medical markings.

Willard, Terry, PhD. *Herbs, Their Clinical Uses: An Easy to Understand Encyclopedic Guide to Herbal & Nutritional Treatment*. Calgary, Alberta, Canada: Wild Rose College of Natural Healing, 1996.
> Dr. Willard is one of the finest herbalists in the West. This book is useful and clearly presented.

INDEX

Note: Page numbers in bold indicate major discussions.

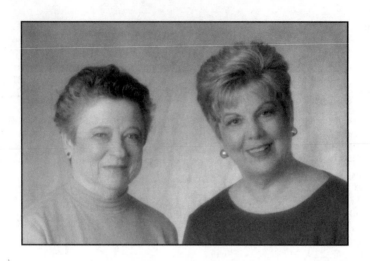

About the Authors

Margaret Smith Peet, ND, is a naturopath with a specialty in Ayurveda. After an early career in music, she turned to editing, working for a number of years with Betty Friedan in preparation of *The Fountain of Age*. In addition to her current book, other writing includes two books and numerous articles for Dr. Vasant Lad. Dr. Peet was a full-time student of Dr. Lad at the Ayurvedic Institute in Albuquerque for five years. She has also studied extensively in the areas of T'ai Chi Chuan, Chinese Herbal Medicine, and Shiatsu. In more recent years, she has been involved in the emerging field of functional medicine. Dr. Peet lives in Maine.

Shoshana Zimmerman, ND, is a naturopath primarily interested in treating three stages of illness using Ayurvedic diagnosis as well as laboratory testing: pre-disease (the stage prior to a diagnosable disease), chronic pain, and chronic illness, combining assessment tools of Ayurveda and Chinese medicine from the East with naturopathic and functional medicine approaches from the West. After early years in the Peace Corps and many years in management, including serving as Assistant Director of a large tertiary care medical center and also as CEO of a manufacturing corporation, Dr. Zimmerman turned to complementary medicine as her main career focus. Dr. Zimmerman also spent five years studying with Dr. Vasant Lad at the Ayurveda Institute in Albuquerque. Her goal is to help people improve the way their body functions through nutrients, food, exercise, stress management, and lifestyle changes. Dr. Zimmerman lives in California's Silicon Valley, where she maintains a private practice in Palo Alto, California.